*Acupuncture as Revolution* offers a trenchant socia[l] traditional Chinese Medicine, and their intersectio[n] health disparities, and medical justice in the Unite[d]

—James Doucet-Battl[e, author of] *Sweetness in the Blood: Race, Risk, and Type 2 Diabetes*

A captivating study of how radical activists, armed with an antidote to heroin withdrawal, battled with elite policymakers over inequities in health and medicine. This story provides insight into the history of the current American opioid epidemic and how acupuncture disrupted the plan. It's a fascinating read for acupuncturists, activists, and readers who enjoy learning about events that impact national public health.

—Jennifer A. M. Stone, senior editor, *Medical Acupuncture*

In America, prior to the 1970s, East Asian medicine and acupuncture were essentially unknown outside of Asian communities. The history and acceptance of this remarkable ancient medicine into mainstream USA is certainly worthy of scholarly research. With her thoughtful, well-researched and beautifully written book, Rachel Pagones has provided a compelling history of the role acupuncture played in the long and continuing struggle for health and racial justice in America.

—Richard Gold, cofounder of Pacific College of Health and Science

*Acupuncture as Revolution* is a timely publication. After the murder of George Floyd, the profession of licensed acupuncturists and the broader integrative health movement are engaging efforts to heal entrenched diversity and equity challenges. The best in the dominant medical industry are seeking to incorporate into their services respect for a broader swath of healthcare determinants. The multiracial experiment that is the United States can seem to be breaking apart. Pagones guides readers into a time and story 50 years ago that adds to the scholarly literature correcting the dominant white rendition of the missions of the Black Panthers and the Young Lords. She shows how, to serve the health of communities broken by racism and intentional neglect, these organizations and their allies in the South Bronx reached outside of accepted practices to fold acupuncture into a remarkable model of community engagement. *Acupuncture as Revolution* provides both acupuncturists and the integrative health movement an origin story that is a remarkable counter to the white privilege with which each is often associated. Rachel Pagones' combination of history, sociology, and science offers signals of what it might take for the dreams of a paradigm shift—from medicine's industrial priorities toward health creation—to actually become the "revolution" promised in her book's title.

—John Weeks, author of the *Integrator Blog* and former editor-in-chief of the *Journal of Alternative and Complementary Medicine*

*Acupuncture as Revolution* is an engaging and timely contribution that sheds new light on acupuncture's radical lineage and its contemporary descendants. In this eye-opening and highly readable history, Pagones restores to their proper place key actors and traditions, from China's barefoot doctors to the Bronx's Young Lords. This book should be read by everyone who cares about acupuncture and alternative movements to promote health.

—Andrew Zitcer, author of *Practicing Cooperation: Mutual Aid beyond Capitalism*

# Acupuncture as Revolution

SUFFERING, LIBERATION, AND LOVE

**Rachel Pagones**

BREVIS PRESS

London

Published by Brevis Press
27 Old Gloucester Street
London
WC1N 3AX

British Library Cataloguing in Publication data
A Catalogue record for this book is available from the British Library

ISBN: 978-1-7399221-0-8 (paperback)
ISBN: 978-1-7399221-1-5 (ebook)

Editing, design, and production by Joanne Shwed, Backspace Ink (www.backspaceink.com)

Cover illustration ©Alfonso Navarro-Reverter

To the memory of my mother,
Dorrie Davenport Pagones

Once or twice in a lifetime,
a man or woman may choose
a radical leaving, having heard
*Lech l'cha*—Go forth.
God disturbs us toward our destiny
by hard events
and by freedom's now urgent voice
which explode and confirm who we are.
—Rabbi Norman Hirsh

# Contents

# List of Acronyms and Abbreviations

| | |
|---|---|
| ACAOM | Accreditation Commission for Acupuncture and Oriental Medicine |
| AIDS | acquired immunodeficiency syndrome |
| AMA | American Medical Association |
| AWB | Acupuncturists Without Borders |
| BAAANA | Black Acupuncture Advisory Association of North America |
| BCD | Board Certified Diplomate in Clinical Social Work |
| BPP | Black Panther Party |
| CCP | Chinese Communist Party |
| CIA | Central Intelligence Agency |
| COINTELPRO | counterintelligence program |
| EIR | Executive Intelligence Review |
| FBI | Federal Bureau of Investigation |
| FDA | Food and Drug Administration |
| GERAC | German Acupuncture Trials |
| HBCU | Historically Black College and University |
| Health/PAC | Health Policy Advisory Center |
| HIV | human immunodeficiency virus |
| HRUM | Health Revolutionary Unity Movement |

| | |
|---|---|
| IBS | irritable bowel syndrome |
| *JCM* | *Journal of Chinese Medicine* |
| LCSW | Licensed Clinical Social Worker |
| MBGC | Madame Binh Graphics Collective |
| NAACP | National Association for the Advancement of Colored People |
| NADA | National Acupuncture Detoxification Association |
| NCCA | National Commission for the Certification of Acupuncture |
| NCCAM | National Center for Complementary and Alternative Medicine |
| NCCAOM | National Certification Commission for Acupuncture and Oriental Medicine |
| NCCIH | National Center for Complementary and Integrative Health |
| NCLC | National Caucus of Labor Committees |
| NIH | National Institutes of Health |
| OCOM | Oregon College of Oriental Medicine |
| POCA | People's Organization of Community Acupuncture |
| PUMC | Peking Union Medical College |
| RICO | Racketeer Influenced and Corrupt Organizations [Act] |
| RNA | Republic of New Afrika |
| SDS | Students for a Democratic Society |
| SHO | Student Health Organization |
| TCM | Traditional Chinese Medicine |
| UCLA | University of California, Los Angeles |
| WCA | Working Class Acupuncture |
| WHO | World Health Organization |
| ZANU | Zimbabwe African National Union |

# Prologue

In April 2018 I was in San Juan, Puerto Rico, to attend a panel discussion at the Colegio de Abogados y Abogadas de Puerto Rico, the Puerto Rico Bar Association. The association is a progressive non-governmental organization, which has taken a strong stand against the death penalty, putting it at odds with the US federal government. The headquarters is also an event venue, often hosting gatherings of progressive organizations. On this occasion, the panel was convened by a group of acupuncturists called Proyecto Salud y Acupuntura para el Pueblo (Health and Acupuncture Project for the People); the topic was "Health, Dignity, and Poverty: A Matter of Human Rights." It was a bright evening, the air still sticky with the day's heat. As dusk fell, the lights did not come on; although electricity had officially been restored to the island, there were still frequent, unexpected outages of unpredictable length. The organizers were prepared though, and soon the generators hummed to life, powering not only light but air conditioning.

Seven months earlier, Hurricane Maria had shredded the island, with 155-mile-per hour winds ripping apart homes, while storm surges and extreme rainfall provoked a lethal combination of coastal flooding and inland flash floods and landslides. No part of the island was spared, with electricity comprehensively knocked out as well as much of the cell phone service. The US government's response, led by President Donald Trump, had been, by its own findings, "chaotic and tragically inadequate," with an official estimate of nearly 3,000 deaths reported one

1

year after the storm.[1] Nonetheless, the president trumpeted the "fantastic job" of his government's response and blamed the island's problems on preexisting conditions, much as a health insurance company in the pre-Affordable Care Act days might have denied treatment to a patient based on their health history. In April 2018, the patient remained in unstable condition. While San Juan, the capital and a tourist destination, came alive with generators during power outages, more remote areas still suffered a lack of basic infrastructure; even in San Juan, people could be seen living in tents on the flat roofs of devastated buildings along the coastline. While death counts were disputed—the initial tally had been recorded as 64—the physical and psychological tolls among residents went undocumented and largely unaddressed.

Against that backdrop, a small coalition of acupuncturists had gathered to offer relief to residents in the form of needling specific points in the ear to reduce pain and, more importantly, to induce calm and alleviate trauma. Acupuncture might seem, of all things, an inadequate response to natural disaster, but there was precedent for the Puerto Rican group's actions, most recently by the organization Acupuncturists Without Borders (AWB), modeled on the physicians' group Médecins Sans Frontières. AWB, in turn, had taken inspiration from the National Acupuncture Detoxification Association (NADA), which had been borne from a program to treat heroin addiction with acupuncture at Lincoln Hospital in the South Bronx of New York in the 1970s. That program—commonly known as Lincoln Detox—had been started by an amalgam of activists, prominently featuring the Young Lords, the group of young revolutionary nationalist Puerto Ricans active in the late 1960s and early 1970s, and spearheaded by two men, Mutulu Shakur and Walter Bosque. Bosque, of Puerto Rican descent, was one of the panelists in San Juan. Sitting next to him was Mario Wexu, a French Canadian who had trained many of the acupuncturists at Lincoln. Bosque and Wexu had spent the previous week in Puerto Rico, giving training to the Puerto Rican acupuncturists and treating hurricane victims. While there were other speakers on the panel, discussing overmedication in the elderly and exploring the link between deaths from the hurricane and poverty, the evening was a reunion of sorts: Along with Bosque and Wexu, the attendees included a handful of the acupuncturists who had worked at Lincoln Hospital in the 1970s and had not seen one another for years. The poster advertising it also seemed like a throwback, illustrated with a cutout from a political poster for the Young Lords, showing a worker with a shovel dug into the earth, a small tree in a pot at his feet, a raised fist clutching a rifle behind him. Shakur was not at the gathering. He was in a federal penitentiary in Victorville, California, serving a 60-year sentence related to revolutionary activities in the 1970s and early 80s. The panel discussion was dedicated to him as cofounder of the acupuncture detoxification clinic at Lincoln Hospital.

Before the panelists began, several speakers stood to honor Shakur's legacy, linking it to the struggle for human rights in Puerto Rico. Wexu and Bosque spoke last, wearing black T-shirts with a raised-fist logo in 70's-era silkscreen style beneath the words "Salud, resistencia" ("Health, resistance"). Each related the story of how acupuncture came to be used at Lincoln Detox and their roles in it. Each telling of the tale had the feeling of grooves worn into an oft-told reminiscence, of a poignant history savored rather than the urgency of the moment. Yet the connection with Puerto Rico's current crisis and with Shakur's spirit of revolutionary change through healing showed the tale to be still relevant. So did impassioned speeches given by organizers and attendees who spoke before the two guest panelists.

Just two weeks earlier, I had been in New York attending another gathering of acupuncturists and other former employees of Lincoln Detox, recounting the same old days but in a different context. This event was held at the New York Society for Ethical Culture; it had been a struggle to get to the building, in a quiet spot just a side street's remove from densely packed crowds assembled for the March for Our Lives protest, a nationwide response to the mass shooting that had killed 17 high school students in Parkland, Florida, the previous month. Inside, the occasion was a memorial service for Dr. Michael Smith, one of the architects of the NADA technique and its chief promoter, who had died in December. The numerous colleagues and family members who paid tribute to him all spoke movingly of the time they shared at Lincoln, performing and promoting acupuncture for drug detox beginning in the 1970s, during times that were hard and volatile. In hindsight, the times also seemed full of warmth and humor—or, perhaps more accurately, of humanity.

Notably, the two reunions did not include any of the same people. Shakur was mentioned once at Smith's memorial, when Carlos Alvarez, who had been with Lincoln Detox from its earliest days, called for a shout-out to the activists who were there from the beginning. When he called Shakur's name, there were cries of "Yes! Yes!" and enthusiastic applause. However, Bosque and others who showed up in Puerto Rico were not there, although they lived in New York. Likewise, Smith was noted only once, tangentially, during the Puerto Rican panel discussion. It seemed odd there was so little connection between the two gatherings—but, as I was to find out later, a schism had occurred between Shakur and Smith just as Lincoln Detox was gaining momentum. That split, based on ideology and practice, would lead to two distinct lineages of acupuncture. Both would be focused on treating addiction and trauma, but one was also determined to change society using acupuncture as a means of revolution.

In a church basement in Portland, Oregon, in June 2018, I listened to another group of acupuncturists fervently debate how to make a better world. They pinpointed socioeconomic inequities and the "white supremacy culture"—the grossly unequal and unjust results of a culture based on favoring white people—as the chief obstacles they needed to overcome. In contrast to the participants in New York and Puerto Rico, most of these acupuncturists were white and too young to have been born in the 1970s. Through the occasional burst of piano playing and the sound of thunderous footsteps overhead—a wedding was taking place on the main floor of the church—there was collective, passionate discussion about how to reach people who were marginalized by society, how to provide acupuncture to them while being sensitive to their needs and trauma, and how to do it affordably. Above all, they argued about how to do it, while negotiating the paradox of being a beneficiary of the very culture you believe is at fault for the marginalization and trauma of the people you want to help. There were no easy answers. But the acupuncturists took heart and inspiration from their "spiritual ancestors," two of whom were Michael Smith and Mutulu Shakur. Clearly there was still a living connection to the events, for better and worse, that began during the turbulent early 1970s and lasted for a decade. Not just grooves in an aging memory, the troubled times, the personal trials, and the techniques of acupuncture as a remedy to social injustice are relevant today. To fully grasp them now requires an understanding of their complex and hard-earned origins.

# Revolutionary Acupuncture

> I remember the first group of UCLA doctors who
> went to China and came back and showed films of
> a horse having acupuncture anesthesia. There was
> sort of a seamless web between barefoot doctors
> and community acupuncture. They were going
> there to refine revolutionary skills. It is a whole
> different thing, such a unique form of idealism—
> that this can be done through the tip of a needle.
>
> —Mark Kleiman, lawyer for Mutulu Shakur

**M**edicine and healthcare in the United States stand at a crossroads. In one direction is integrative medicine, an evolving approach embedded in numerous major universities. Acupuncture, which was once classified "alternative medicine" and then "complementary and alternative medicine" now falls under the umbrella of "traditional, complementary, and integrative medicine." Revolutionary acupuncture movements have emphasized community treatments, while integrative medicine is enthusiastically exploring the potential of group visits, particularly in underserved communities. In this sense, acupuncture seems poised to fit into a new niche in integrative medicine: that of an inexpensive, low-tech, easily transportable therapy that can be delivered in a group setting to marginalized people. Indeed, as this chapter will show, that is not a new use of acupuncture; what is new is the possibility of its acceptance as such within a mainstream healthcare system.

At the same time, acupuncture's identity is precarious. The once-alluring ring of the word "Oriental," a central component of the name of many colleges and organizations, has become an embarrassment. The profession's association with a privileged white clientele is frustrating to many acupuncturists, even as they find it necessary to court that demographic to pay off weighty student debt. In popular culture, acupuncture has been associated since the 1970s with the counterculture—a "hippie" accoutrement—or is portrayed as an activity of the white "worried well," sometimes parodied in literature and film.[1] More recently, it may be heard of in the context of opioid addiction as an alternative therapy for pain relief, or even as treatment for addiction itself. But, as a key part of Chinese medicine, acupuncture is far more than a trendy modality or a specific therapy for addiction or pain. Nor can it be properly perceived as an ancient system, either preserved through time or adapted to local cultural demands. Anthropologist Mei Zhan, in *Other-Worldly*, presents alternative ways of perceiving traditional Chinese medicine as it is transmitted across boundaries, a process she calls "worlding." Zhan likens the process to a flow of water creating geographic formations through time. Extending the analogy, the daily effects may be imperceptible, but it is the accumulated everyday encounters "mundane and extraordinary at the same time" that shape momentous changes.[2]

Zhan's concept of worlding helps to explain historic shifts that were significant to the story of revolutionary acupuncture and continue to shape its course. A "wave of institutionalization" in the 1950s, which led to the standardization of the medicine known as Traditional Chinese Medicine (TCM) under Mao Zedong's direction, resulted in the export of acupuncture to Africa and other colonized regions as part of the bid of the Chinese Communist Party (CCP) to lead a world revolution. China's efforts in Africa and elsewhere strongly influenced the politics of revolutionary acupuncturists in the 1970s. But activist acupuncturists today live in a world shaped by a subsequent wave of "dense translocal encounters" during which the flow of TCM shifted from poor rural populations in developing countries to relatively prosperous populations in the developed world. At the same time, preventive medicine in the context of TCM was redefined, from basic primary care to mind-body wellness, from a necessity to a middle-class accessory. And one cannot just travel to China to recover the old ways; as Zhan explains, a hip California lifestyle is as desired in Shanghai as it is in Palo Alto.[3]

This explanation helps to account for the reason acupuncture may still be perceived in the United States as primarily an option for the white and the wealthy—despite its use in underserved communities, from refugee camps to free clinics for older adults to the sites of natural disasters, and despite an increasingly vocal contingent of acupuncturists of color.[4] Another reason, emphasized by the community acupuncturists in Portland, Oregon, is the structure of the educational system, which is expensive and arguably based in a narrative of and for affluent white people.[5] The educational structure is linked by some scholars to the colonization of indigenous medicine (used by and subsumed within biomedicine) as well as systemic racism affecting access to education and to complementary and alternative care.[6] The perception of such factors within acupuncture and integrative medicine is a strong motivator for change today.

"Worlding" sees changes affected by, and effecting, the intersections of biomedicine, scientific research, professionalization, regional and global politics, and cultural evolution. But, too, they are contingent on the everyday encounter. The encounters of the history I tell in the following pages—between revolutionary acupuncturists, the people to whom they provided acupuncture, and society—are significant to healthcare and racial justice activists today. I believe the potential exists for acupuncturists, such as the ones in Puerto Rico and Portland, to add their everyday actions, extraordinary and mundane, to the re-creation of a more inclusive and integrated healthcare. The historic influences that helped propel them to the present moment, however, have been largely unexplored and unrecognized.

## Why Acupuncture?

The quiet insertion of fine needles into a sitting or prone person's body in order to rebalance a perceived disharmony seems an unlikely revolutionary tactic. It seems still less so in the context of the 1960s and 70s, an historically turbulent time in which guns, bombs, protests, police brutality, and extrajudicial killings were all deployed on the field of revolutionary politics in the United States. Yet in the events that followed the forceful takeover of a New York City municipal hospital involving nunchakus and shurikens or throwing stars (although the weapons were not used), a dedicated cadre of acupuncturists was formed. This group was committed to upholding the principle that the ability to choose and control one's healthcare is a basic human right. Their commitment was to poor, marginalized, and oppressed people; in the South Bronx and Harlem during that time, where the acupuncture cadre honed its skills and trained young recruits, those people were mostly Black Americans and Puerto Ricans. The group took the form, as many movements in the 1970s did, of a collective, which, while providing acupuncture treatments to the community, also trained some community members to perform acupuncture. When the collective was broken up by the City of New York, its members created a college to provide formal acupuncture training, and when that college was shut down by the Federal Bureau of Investigation (FBI), some of the remaining acupuncturists opened another. After the second college's demise, largely due to financial reasons, a handful of its former adherents continued to offer acupuncture to the community from the basements of New York City churches.

The New York City collective formed the first revolutionary acupuncture movement in the United States. I call this movement revolutionary detox acupuncture in recognition of its central goal of combating heroin addiction in the community. (When applied to an individual, the process of combating addiction was known as drug detoxification, shortened to detox.) Revolutionary detox acupuncture, in common with many youthful movements of the 1960s, was rooted in revolutionary politics.[7] These roots in turn were embedded in circumstances both local and global. Locally, heroin addiction and appallingly inadequate healthcare were two of the factors ravaging communities in the South Bronx of New York City; globally, the era was defined by the international student protests of 1968, the Vietnam War, and liberation movements in Africa, Asia, and Latin America. The politics underlying revolutionary detox acupuncture were strongly influenced by three related phenomena: the loose collection of left-wing movements known as the New Left[8]; Maoism; and the CCP's policy of medical diplomacy in what was then known as the Third World, particularly in Africa.

Revolutionary detox acupuncture, like much of the New Left, identified with a spate of successful and ongoing liberation wars by formerly colonized African and Southeast Asian nations as well as the Cuban revolution. Its anticolonialist/anticapitalist stance belonged to the view known as Third World Marxism or Third World socialism, which was also embraced by the most prominent Black Power and revolutionary nationalist groups of the 1960s and early 1970s, the Black Panther Party (BPP) and the Young Lords.[9] This view perceived racism and its insidious effects within the United States as a form of domestic colonization inextricably tied to Western imperialism and capitalism. It saw the most oppressed people—Karl Marx's lumpenproletariat—as the best-situated revolutionary actors.[10]

However, a unique element of revolutionary detox acupuncture was its focus on "chemical warfare" as a manifestation of US imperialism and corrupt capitalism. By this analysis, capitalist powers, including the US government and pharmaceutical companies, conspired to push heroin into ghetto communities, such as Harlem and the South Bronx, to effectively tranquilize the residents, who were primarily African American and Puerto Rican. As a result, the people would not have the inner resources to fight back against racial oppression. Radical activists connected this analysis to Central Intelligence Agency (CIA) involvement in heroin production and trade in Southeast Asia, which was uncovered by scholarly investigation and resultant congressional hearings in the early 1970s.[11] The argument was not unique to revolutionary acupuncturists—the Young Lords also embraced it, and it had earlier roots among leftist thinkers and the Black Power movement—but it became a raison d'être for their leader Mutulu Shakur.[12]

Like most of its contemporary political movements, revolutionary detox acupuncture did not survive beyond the 1970s. From its remains, though, came the second US revolutionary acupuncture movement; it was embodied in First World Acupuncture, an acupuncture college and clinic established in Harlem in the early 1980s. First World Acupuncture sought to maintain the vision and praxis of revolutionary detox acupuncture without the political engagement. Although its founders maintained their political ideals, they did not convey them to the students or clients of the clinic, instead focusing on the themes of healthcare as a human right and the right of Black and Latinx people to learn Chinese medicine and other indigenous medical traditions.

While revolutionary detox acupuncture both imagined and advertised acupuncture as an overtly political form of healing, First World Acupuncture purveyed it first and foremost as a tool of racial and social justice for marginalized communities. This vision for acupuncture, incorporated into a formal college, made it unique in North American acupuncture education until the creation of POCA Tech, the college founded by the People's Organization of Community Acupuncture, in 2014. The politics underlying First World Acupuncture remained fundamental to the existence of the college and clinic. However, for the very practical reason that survival as an overtly revolutionary institution would have been untenable after the demise of revolutionary detox acupuncture and in the political climate of the 1980s, the political aspect remained unspoken. First World Acupuncture fell apart after a few short, intense years, unable to maintain its coherence against financial and logistical dictates as well as personal demands as its members aged out of youth. Its vision and goals seemed lost to time. But in the early years of the twenty-first century, a third form of revolutionary acupuncture arose.

Liberation Acupuncture—a praxis formed of a body of thought derived from liberation theology plus the practice of community acupuncture—was formed three decades after First World Acupuncture in a profoundly different historical moment. Gone were the militant tendencies, the revolutionary rhetoric, and the countercultural iconoclasms that marked activism in the 1960s and 70s. Nonetheless, the year 2011, when Liberation Acupuncture began taking shape, was also defined by great social divisions. The Occupy movement, which began on Wall Street and spread globally, was an outraged response to the socioeconomic chasm that had opened between the world's top earners—the so-called 1 percent—and the rest of humanity. The movement was informed by the Great Recession of 2007 to 2009, which exposed the complicity of the international banking industry in leveraging the modest wealth of ordinary workers to its own great advantage. When the mortgage industry collapsed and the bulk of the risk fell on the worker rather than the banks, existing socioeconomic and racial disparities were exposed and widened. In 2013, as Liberation Acupuncture continued its formation, the racial justice movement Black Lives Matter was founded, sharpening the focus on persistent anti-Black racism. And within healthcare, the concept of trauma-informed care, which has its roots in the treatment of Vietnam War veterans, took root as a new paradigm in public health and mental health services.[13]

Liberation Acupuncture does not exercise revolutionary politics in the mode of 1960s and 70s activists. Its broad goal is to help right the socially engendered illnesses of people living outside the privileges of the dominant culture. Like its predecessors, it promulgates the principles of choice and control of healthcare as human rights. Based in Portland, Oregon, the movement has formed a cooperative called POCA and opened a low-cost college, POCA Tech. The community acupuncture model of low-priced treatments given in a group setting was inspired by the revolutionary detox acupuncture movement of the 1970s, and POCA takes moral inspiration from some of the founders of that movement. Liberation Acupuncture consciously echoes the concepts of liberation theology and liberation psychology but also of the Black liberation movement. It shares with the earlier revolutionary acupuncture movements the core tenet that disease can only be understood in the context of socioeconomic forces. And it is motivated by a fundamental disagreement with the racial and socioeconomic inequities of society. Because of these radical similarities and because Liberation Acupuncture views acupuncture as a means to promote and engender social change, I contend that it belongs to the lineage of revolutionary acupuncture movements.

These three movements join other examples of radical activism to combat social and healthcare inequities; the Black Panthers and the Young Lords (both of whom were closely associated with the early formation of revolutionary detox acupuncture) also used direct action to influence, improve, or create community healthcare programs. Recently historians have shown these efforts to be significant aspects of the groups' revolutionary politics and to have had a lasting impact, even though the movements themselves did not last.[14] Revolutionary acupuncture therefore raises important questions: Why address these deeply embedded societal challenges with acupuncture? What is the legacy of the revolutionary acupuncture movement of the 1970s? And, ultimately, can the practice of acupuncture within a revolutionary framework meaningfully influence underlying social conditions?

## Global Revolution and Maoism

The origins of revolutionary detox acupuncture were steeped in a sense of global struggle and change. In the 1960s and early 1970s, as youthful American activists of color perceived the shackles of colonial rule falling from countries in Africa, Asia, and Latin America, they identified their own oppression, ideals, and goals with those battles for liberation around the world.[15] The analysis that racism at home was a mirror of colonialism abroad was central to the activism that Max Elbaum labels the New Communist Movement—an aspect of the New Left—and, particularly, to activists of color.[16] The latter included the Black Panthers and the Young Lords. Those groups did not conceive of the concept though; it began in the early 1960s with Black radical thinkers who saw isolation and exploitation of African Americans as a parallel of imperialism in the Third World.[17]

Global struggle was seen primarily through the lens of Maoism, which had become the dominant form of Marxist-Leninist theory among New Left and liberation activists who were mainly influenced by the interpretations of leaders including Mao Zedong, Fidel Castro, and Che Guevara.[18] Around the world, Mao's theories and the actions of the CCP had tremendous influence during this period. Historian Julia Lovell coined the term "high Maoism" to encompass the Great Leap Forward, the Sino-Soviet split, and the Cultural Revolution—an era lasting from the late 1950s to the mid-1970s, the time of "Mao's revolution in its most expansive phase."[19]

One of the key locales to which the revolution expanded was Africa. Particularly following the Sino-Soviet split—the ideological and political rupture between China and the USSR, after which the two powers vied for the title of world leader of the revolution—Mao and his CCP nurtured relations with African nations ready to engage in revolution. The CCP's focus reflected a vision of Africa's place in the world revolution it sought to lead but also its own struggle for influence in global diplomacy.[20] While the CCP gave both money and military training to African countries, medical cooperation or "medical diplomacy" became one of its most important and influential strategies.[21] Among the medical resources sent to Africa were workers trained in rural healthcare, including barefoot doctors—young people from suitably revolutionary backgrounds who were trained in basic principles and techniques of both biomedicine and TCM, including herbal medicine and acupuncture.[22] For instance, in 1964, China began building a healthcare system based on the barefoot doctor model in the nascent United Republic of Tanzania. Other African nations where acupuncture was deployed were Mali, Mauritania, Sudan, Zambia, and Zanzibar.[23]

# The Barefoot Doctors

The barefoot doctor concept—if not an exact replica of the model used in China—was to become an unexpectedly influential form of Maoist medical diplomacy well beyond Africa. The concept of preventative medicine, making use of indigenous knowledge and simple techniques, packaged in the form of a humble, community-spirited paraprofessional and ready to transport to remote rural areas, impressed not only revolutionaries but prominent Western medical doctors and public health organizations.[24] Some physicians had traveled to China as early as 1971, the year before Nixon's historic visit; after the United States and China formally opened relations, other curious physicians as well as radical activists—including members of the BPP and revolutionary detox acupuncture—toured China, where they witnessed acupuncture treatments and learned more about the barefoot doctors. The visitors were undoubtedly given a selective view of Chinese society and healthcare; however, their impressions were more than romantic visions of a harder truth couched in propaganda. The barefoot doctors were in fact quite effective in improving healthcare in rural China, and the model adapted well to Africa.[25] Additionally, medical and technology historian Mary Augusta Brazelton writes of the "global popularization of Chinese public health" in the 1960s and 70s, noting that China used not only medical aid to developing countries but invitations to international doctors and scholars to advertise its success in public health—and the diplomacy worked in both developed and developing nations. Inasmuch as China "promoted its system of rural medical care as a model for the future of global health governance," Mao created an international, rather than a provincial, impression, one that extended all the way to the World Health Organization (WHO).[26]

The Declaration of Alma-Ata in 1978 was a WHO treatise on primary healthcare that established health as a fundamental human right. The declaration stated that health was tied to socioeconomic well-being and that the existence of vast health inequalities between populations of richer and poorer was unacceptable and of universal concern. Notably, it also affirmed that "the people have the right and duty to participate individually and collectively in the planning and implementation of their health care."[27] The barefoot doctor initiative is now considered one of the primary forces behind the WHO's ideological shift that led to Alma-Ata.[28]

## Everywhere in the News

While they did not make the media splash that acupuncture eventually did, the barefoot doctors were everywhere in the news from the late 1960s through the early 1970s. From 1968 to 1973, nearly 50,000 newspaper articles were published on the barefoot doctors across North America—from San Francisco to Palm Beach; from Minneapolis to Honolulu; from Jackson, Mississippi, to Louisville, Kentucky; from Asbury Park, New Jersey, to Chula Vista, California.[29] (They enjoyed a yet more dramatic rise in popularity in China, with their number more than doubling, to more than one million, during the same period.)[30] Prior to Nixon's visit, some articles were derogatory, even scathing, about everything from the political theory behind the program to the barefoot doctors' clothing. One such article, "'Barefoot Doctors' Replace Practitoners [sic] in Red China," published in the *Lansing State Journal* in 1968, began: "Except for specialists, the practitioner of Western medicine has virtually disappeared from China." The article claimed the doctors of China were "abandoning their classrooms, their instruments and their libraries in a movement that can only set back scientific progress for political expediency." The content and tone of the piece, filled with inflammatory language such as "appalling" and "heart-breaking," reflects the fervent anti-Communist sentiment of the era.[31]

Later articles, however, were increasingly positive in tone. A 1971 report in the *Palm Beach Post-Times* focused on the benefits of making healthcare available and affordable to the masses. It began: "China's 'new medicine' is making it possible for the nation's 600 million peasants to have medical treatment never available before. The cost is less than 50 U.S. cents a year." It emphasized the barefoot doctors' education and training and admired the well-equipped commune facilities, in stark contrast to the 1968 excoriation. Yet, despite praising the blend of Chinese and Western medicine used, the article mentioned acupuncture only once and with little confidence. After noting all barefoot doctors were trained in the practice, it observed, "Acupuncture is an ancient method of inserting needles into a patient's nerve centers to relieve pain. Western medicine holds it to be quackery."[32]

By 1973, there was still extensive interest in the barefoot doctors, aided by the opening of relations after Nixon's visit a year earlier, which enabled official government tours during which the Chinese government was keen to advertise one of the key components of its modern health policy.[33] Press reports were by now laudatory. An article in the *Asbury Park Press* carrying the headline "China's 'Barefoot Doctors' Produce Medical Revolution" was emphatically positive about both acupuncture and the barefoot doctors. Its comments on public health reflect the far-reaching success of Mao's medical diplomacy:

> China startled the medical world with breakthroughs using acupuncture as a treatment for ailments and as anesthesia for major surgery. But perhaps more important in Chinese medicine today is the development of hundreds of thousands of paramedics in the rice roots areas of China called "barefoot doctors." Some of the most impressive achievements in modern China have been accomplished through the use of these barefoot doctors who have brought medical care to the farthest reaches of the country and who have been in the vanguard of public health and preventive medicine.[34]

The article emphasized the affordability and availability of medicine made possible to all citizens through the program, presumably its most revolutionary aspect from an American point of view. It also highlighted the facts that the practitioners had ongoing training and made outside referrals to fully trained medical doctors for serious conditions, the lack of which were bemoaned by the 1968 article. A further 1973 article, from *The Greenville News* in South Carolina, reported on a government visit including eight American physicians. Headlined "China's 'Barefoot Doctors' Win Praise from 2 U.S. Physicians," the report claimed the American doctors were not only impressed by China's program but were considering ways to apply it in the United States. One of the physicians, an assistant medical director at the State Department, was quoted as saying, "Many U.S. doctors are spinning their wheels doing lots of things they don't have to do. If we could make use of something like the barefoot doctors, American health care would be better off."[35]

The State Department doctor was not alone in his opinion. Other figures from both the medical community and academia, who had been invited to China during the rush of interest from both sides surrounding Nixon's 1972 visit, returned deeply impressed by the advances in healthcare they witnessed. Moreover, they wrote about their impressions in journals and symposia, spreading the word beyond the credulous public to the more skeptical scientific community in such prestigious establishment publications as the *New England Journal of Medicine* and the *Journal of the American Medical Association*. One of the first doctors to tour China in the 1970s was Victor W. Sidel, head of the Department of Social Medicine at Montefiore Hospital in the Bronx, an institution tied to Lincoln Hospital through its relationship with Albert Einstein College of Medicine (discussed in Chapter 1). Sidel took a highly favorable view of the barefoot doctors in an article for the *New England Journal of Medicine*. His introductory disclaimer describes the mindset of a significant minority of healthcare professionals at that time: "My bias that there is much that needs improvement in the American health-care system—and in American society in general—unquestionably led me to look with friendly interest on a system of social and health services that has produced almost unbelievable progress in 22 years."[36]

Another doctor who was on the trip with Sidel, in September 1971, Paul Dudley White—a prominent cardiologist who had been President

Dwight D. Eisenhower's personal physician—observed that the Chinese were ahead of Americans when it came to the delivery of healthcare.[37] Again, his was not an isolated impression. It was, in fact, a critical insight shared by medical doctors, social scientists, and revolutionary political activists who had been given a glimpse of China's healthcare system, and they all attributed much of that system's success to the barefoot doctor program. The emphasis on using community personnel and collective action in nonprofessional delivery of primary healthcare to deprived areas was not only a medical matter but a sociopolitical one.[38] The ramifications were extensive for all invested in changing their particular part of the "system," but perhaps most of all for revolutionary healthcare activists who were promulgating the tenet that health must be understood as a function of socioeconomic and political forces— and, therefore, that social, economic, and political change was necessary.

In China, the CCP also used the press to promote the barefoot doctors, and its language and slogans advertised the image and spirit of young revolutionary forces. Frequently described as "newly emerged things," the barefoot doctors were said to be armed with "one silver needle and a bunch of herbs," i.e., the basic tools of acupuncture and Chinese herbal medicine. The simplicity of the image was powerful, although in fact the practitioners were as (or more) likely to use a stethoscope and prescribe Western antibiotics as they were to employ traditional methods.[39]

Both the Chinese and Western press, likely for different reasons, left out some important features of the barefoot doctor initiative. One was the selection criteria, which included both an aptitude for learning and the correct political background, i.e., being from the poor and lower-middle peasant classes and displaying sufficient revolutionary fervor.[40] Candidates were ideally graduates of middle school (roughly equal to a junior high school education in the United States) and were often chosen personally by brigade secretaries for their intelligence. While candidates could be any age, younger people aged 17-20, who were old enough to be school graduates but young enough to be unmarried and therefore less encumbered, were preferred; the average age of barefoot doctors at one commune was given as 23.[41] Females were supposed to be equally represented, a tremendous change from a system in which women's health had been woefully neglected due to cultural taboos that precluded, for instance, even the exposure of an arm for a vaccine. While in practice the ratio of females to males was somewhat less than 50-50, the image of young female barefoot doctors was often used for revolutionary propaganda posters in the 1970s.[42]

Knowledge about the barefoot doctors made its way through various conduits to the activists in New York who became involved in revolutionary detox acupuncture. In Chinatown they purchased booklets featuring the barefoot doctors published by the People's Liberation Army Publishing House.[43] As mentioned earlier, a few traveled to China on trips sponsored by the Chinese government, during which they heard about the barefoot doctors and may have seen some of them in action. Many, however, seemed to have absorbed some knowledge of the barefoot doctors without really knowing where it came from, and the term itself, with its image of a humble yet skilled servant of the people, may have exerted the most powerful grip of all. (In fact, the "barefoot doctors" wore shoes but were so called to emphasize their solidarity with the peasants who often toiled barefoot in the fields.)[44]

The revolutionary acupuncturists' impressions were varied. One former student of First World Acupuncture said she was drawn to study acupuncture partly because of "the idea that it was a low-tech medicine, inspired by barefoot medicine practice of the Vietnam war."[45] She distinctly remembered Vietnam veterans speaking of barefoot doctors they witnessed practicing during the war. On the other hand, Franklin Apfel, who began working at Lincoln Hospital after graduating from medical school at Columbia University and became the first medical director of its acupuncture program, recalled a book as the source of his knowledge of barefoot doctors. Interestingly, the book Apfel cited, *Where There Is No Doctor: A Village Health Care Handbook*, does not mention barefoot doctors.[46] It is, as the subtitle suggests, a practical guide to providing medical care in places without many resources. Apfel remembered *Where There Is No Doctor* as an inspiration to many of his colleagues, and indeed the book's philosophy and practical approach fit with the reputation the barefoot doctor program had already gained as a low-cost solution built around easily available indigenous medicines. Apfel's conflation of the handbook—which sold over three million copies—with the concept of barefoot doctors suggests the extent to which the latter had percolated into the consciousness of radical physicians as well as political revolutionaries.

In fact, the manual widely used by China's barefoot doctors is similar in some key respects to *Where There Is No Doctor*. Both set out core primary-care principles including hygiene and prevention and then describe diagnosis and simple treatment of specific conditions. Both discuss family planning. The Chinese manual also features sections on Chinese differential diagnosis, acupuncture, and herbal medicine, with the latter taking the last 391 pages of the 942-page book, including sketches of the plants and details of where to find them.[47]

The BPP, which had a great interest in community healthcare, had also traveled to China, on two trips from 1971 to 1972. During the first trip, in September and October of 1971, BPP leader Huey Newton met Chinese premier Chou En-lai; reportedly, the second visit of a contingent of Blank Panthers was agreed at this time.[48] The second trip took place in March 1972. It consisted of 18 people, among them BPP members and one of their lawyers, and lasted seven weeks. The BPP was deeply involved in community initiatives to bring better healthcare to Black Americans, and the party included Dr. Tolbert Small, a medical doctor who had treated the radical intellectual Angela Davis while she was held in the Marin County Jail in 1970.[49] Small observed acupuncture for the first time in China, where he and the others received some rudimentary training and learned to needle themselves; he noted this was also how the barefoot doctors learned needling technique.[50] Small continued to use acupuncture in his Oakland, California, clinic after returning to the United States and, although he was not a BPP member, he was a doctor to the Black Panthers. The impressions of Small or other BPP members from that trip may have made their way to people involved at Lincoln.

# The Ding County Experiment and Professionalism

The barefoot doctor program was contemporary with the origins of revolutionary detox acupuncture. Yet an earlier development in the transformation of healthcare in China may also have influenced the movement, although less directly. Medical historian Sean Hsiang-Lin Lei emphasizes its role in defining the importance of community-controlled healthcare in poor rural areas, while both Fang and the public health historian Liping Bu draw a straight line from the event to implementation of the barefoot doctors.[51] The development was the Ding County experiment of the early 1930s, a trial in affordable rural healthcare controlled by the community. Its architect Chen Zhiqian had trained at the famous Peking Union Medical College (PUMC) and thus held a position at the peak of medical professionalism. Yet Chen—who was influenced by John B. Grant, a key figure in the development of a public health system in China—held some iconoclastic views on professionalism.[52] He wrote that rural China should not depend on experts for its medical needs and, moreover, that the employment of doctors and nurses in rural healthcare should be avoided when possible. Chen's rationale was based on three premises: First, the basic needs of rural healthcare were generally limited and simple enough that doctors and nurses were not needed; second, the high cost of professional help was unaffordable to rural communities; and third, as medical training was a product of the West or Japan, its applicability to China's needs was questionable. Crucially, Chen also held that, because of the government's failure to take responsibility for public health, healthcare should be a collective enterprise. His model was a community-based healthcare movement.[53]

By all accounts, the Ding County experiment was a success. An affordable, effective healthcare system was built over the course of three years. It also became a highly influential model after its results were unveiled at China's National Conference on Rural Reconstruction in 1934. A key feature of Ding County was its divergence from the prevailing model at the time. To the extent the government had been involved in rural healthcare, its approach was top down rather than community based.[54] Furthermore, it was often Western missionary doctors who were assigned to rural areas.[55] Despite their best intentions, whether urban Chinese physicians or missionary medics, these doctors had no intrinsic understanding of the community or its needs.[56]

While New York City of the 1970s and rural China of the 1930s are not direct parallels, their healthcare needs bore key similarities. The South Bronx, a particularly poor area, was in dire need of effective healthcare, yet much of it—for instance, primary care and prevention and prenatal care—could arguably have been handled by trained lay people from the community rather than medical professionals.[57] Such professionals as were available were outsiders, on two levels: The main provider of healthcare in the South Bronx was Lincoln Hospital, and any doctor there was an outsider to the community. Beginning with the Affiliation Program of the 1960s and 70s (discussed in Chapter 1), most of Lincoln's doctors were residents and interns from New York's Albert Einstein College of Medicine or Columbia University's medical college—mainly upper-middle class, mainly white, mainly male, and raised far from the poverty surrounding Lincoln Hospital. Prior to that, Lincoln's doctors had been non-US citizens: foreign medical students or young MDs whom it was easier for the struggling hospital to attract but who had even less invested in the community than American medical students. Moreover, many of them struggled with colloquial English, further alienating the community.[58] Medical provision in New York's public hospitals, and the South Bronx in particular, then, was certainly a top-down system, engineered and staffed by professionals and outsiders, with little understanding of, or ability to deal with, the community's basic healthcare needs.

The matter of professionalism also became a crux of dispute between the hospital and community. As both Fang and the sociologist Paul Root Wolpe have noted, medical practitioners formulate and strengthen their group identity by constraining competition from other social groups with an interest in healthcare.[59] Competition from other groups is effectively limited by the professionalization of medicine. The success of the barefoot doctors was possible in part because the Chinese government could, and did, limit competition from other groups, including folk healers and, to some extent, professional physicians.[60] However, particularly in the West, the power struggle between the proponents of acupuncture and the dominant biomedical paradigm remains an ongoing and lopsided battle.[61]

In summary, the barefoot doctors were a widely hailed phenomenon in the early 1970s, and young people interested in a radical approach to improving medical care for the poor of New York City became aware of and were inspired by it. To revolutionaries, the barefoot doctors were a compelling part of Maoism and fit with their analysis of their own communities' health needs. The barefoot doctors' use of acupuncture and herbal medicine was particularly well advertised by the Chinese government and was a significant component of its attractiveness to Westerners. In addition, although New York City might seem the antithesis of the Chinese countryside, the test applied to rural parts of China was equally applicable to North America's second largest city: whether the basic needs of poor people without access to healthy living conditions or adequate healthcare from the existing medical system could be met by community-based, nonprofessional, people's doctors trained in rudimentary medicine or indigenous methods.

## Countercultural Influence

The counterculture was a backbeat to leftist movements from the mid-1960s to the mid-1970s. Although Theodore Roszak, whose seminal work on the topic was published in 1969, seems to define the US counterculture as a phenomenon of white people, distancing white radicals from the "exploited masses of the Third World" and their revolutionary movements, the reality proved more complex.[62] There is evidence the counterculture had both intangible and practical influences on revolutionaries of color. For example, one member of the Young Lords described Woodstock and other events during the summer of 1969 as inspiring idealistic youth of many ethnicities to work together for universal justice, while sociologist Alondra Nelson writes of the influence of both the Freedom Summer initiative of 1964 and San Francisco's "Summer of Love" in establishing the model of free health clinics adopted by the Black Panthers.[63] The model also clearly influenced the Lincoln Detox clinic, which would become the first clinic using acupuncture to combat drug addiction in the United States and the birthplace of revolutionary detox acupuncture.[64] Countercultural ideologies surrounding concepts of health certainly influenced the increasing popularity of acupuncture as an East Asian holistic healing modality in the 1970s.[65] And in some cases those ideologies merged with political beliefs held by revolutionaries; for instance, in relating Mao's interpretation of dialectical materialism to the principles of Chinese medicine.[66]

## Acupuncture: Perception and Reception

Acupuncture enjoyed something of a meteoric rise in popularity among certain sectors of the American public around the opening of US-China relations in 1972. Prior to the 1970s, most practitioners of Chinese medicine were herbalists practicing in Chinese American communities (although their clientele was often multiethnic).[67] As their unlicensed businesses were subject to punitive measures, some even became licensed chiropractors to achieve professional legitimacy; others encouraged their children to enter biomedicine as a more reliable career path.[68] Acupuncture was not much used and in some cases was denigrated; historian Tamara Venit Shelton describes publications produced by biomedical professionals and Chinese American social workers in the 1960s and 70s that correlated poverty and poor outcomes with Chinese immigrants' use of traditional therapies—including acupuncture.[69]

The most common narrative, among both scholars and contemporary acupuncturists, of how interest in acupuncture outside of Asian communities suddenly swelled cites as a watershed event an article written by James Reston for the New York Times, published on July 26, 1971. Reston, a Pulitzer Prize-winning journalist who was close to National

Security Advisor Henry Kissinger, had traveled to China planning to meet Kissinger but was felled by acute appendicitis. Reston underwent surgery at the Anti-Imperialist Hospital—formerly PUMC, China's most prestigious medical school, which was founded by the Rockefeller Foundation in 1916. After the surgery Reston experienced bloating and pain and was treated successfully with acupuncture needles and the application of a warming herb, a practice known as moxibustion. He wrote eloquently about his experience, including astute observations of the politics of medicine in China, in his *Times* piece.[70] The newspaper followed with an article by Jane Brody in December 1971, describing a demonstration by a Chinese acupuncturist at a meeting of the New York State Society of Anesthesiology. Brody's take was noncommittal; she concluded that the placebo effect had played a possible role and that large placebo-controlled trials were needed before passing judgment.[71]

Many of the flood of subsequent media accounts were less measured than Brody's. They also tended to align acupuncture with a privileged white world—quite the opposite of its earlier associations.[72] A lengthy color piece in the *Los Angeles Times*—written after the first California state bill legalizing acupuncture was passed in 1972—said that acupuncture had "become *de rigeur* [sic] in canape colloquies." It went on to state,

> By now, most of the Western world must be familiar with James Reston's postoperative needle therapy in Peking as well as those exotic acupuncture charts festooned with potbellied, near-naked Chinamen, who are pocked with points and lines and numbers and incomprehensible names like "The Arm Absolute Yin (Circulation-Sex) Meridian.[73]

The article uses a playful and sometimes mocking tone, making use of Orientalisms and referring to "lady doctors" but also striving for some degree of balance by presenting anecdotes of success and comments from MDs making an earnest attempt to be open-minded.

It comes out in favor of acupuncture in the end—"by most any phase of the moon, it works." The article's style and tone may appear abrasive, even offensive, today. However, to paraphrase Mary Augusta Brazelton in describing science historian Sigrid Schmalzer's approach to using propaganda as an historical source, this kind of reporting may be best understood not for its face value but for what it tells us of the experience of people as they lived through the era, and of the understandings and concerns of those who produced the report.[74]

There were numerous concerns, some of which were taken up by scientific and medical researchers. Although acupuncture research in the United States was virtually nonexistent before 1970, by 1974 it made up about 20 percent of the world scientific community's output on the subject.[75] Yet an Orientalist suspicion lingered; an editorial in *Science*, the journal of the American Association for the Advancement of Science, began, "By now, the scarcely veiled thought that acupuncture is some kind of a hoax has lifted, and most Western scientists who have had contact with *men who constitute the closest thing available to an authority on the subject* are convinced that acupuncture works—*in China*."[76] [Emphasis added.] In the intervening years, nonetheless, scientific studies have been extremely important for the acceptance and development of acupuncture in the United States and elsewhere. Indeed, the project of getting traditional Chinese medicine to conform to Western science was in the making well before the 1970s, as Chapter 2 will illustrate.

## Asian American Involvement

This book does not cover the history of acupuncture in the United States prior to 1970, and it does not encompass the history of Chinese medicine in the United States as experienced by Asian American immigrants. Readers who wish to know more of those histories may want to start with Tamara Venit Shelton's *Herbs and Roots: A History of Chinese Doctors in the American Medical Marketplace* and Mei Zhan's *Other-Worldly: Making Chinese Medicine through Transnational*

*Frames.* Revolutionary detox acupuncture did have a significant connection to Asian American radical activism, though. Its leader Mutulu Shakur was close to Yuri Kochiyama, the Japanese American activist who would introduce him to acupuncture. Tatsuo Hirano, another Japanese American organizer who became a revolutionary acupuncturist, met Shakur through Kochiyama and another political connection, Nobuko Miyamoto.[77] Hirano was also close to Shin'ya Ono, a member of the Weatherman, the militant revolutionary entity that preceded the Weather Underground. Many Japanese American radicals had experienced racism through the internment of their families during the Second World War; they were deeply influenced by the civil rights and Black Power movements and identified with the struggles against anti-Black racism.[78]

## Structure of the Book

This chapter has introduced three movements using acupuncture as a means of revolution: revolutionary detox acupuncture, First World Acupuncture, and Liberation Acupuncture. It has situated them in the context of radical healthcare activism as well as revolutionary politics beginning in the 1960s and 1970s and has laid out the diverse influences leading young political revolutionaries to focus on acupuncture.

The rest of the book is structured largely along chronological lines, beginning with a background of the South Bronx and Lincoln Hospital in the early 1970s. Chapter 1 describes the appalling conditions in the South Bronx, leading to record rates of heroin addiction, and analyzes the political and economic ecosystems allowing fires to rage out of control, devastating neighborhoods. It probes the perceptions and theories of healthcare activists involved at Lincoln, from hospital workers to radicalized young doctors to community members and revolutionary movements. It explores the concept of medical empires, the critical issue of community-worker control, and the controversial matter of professionalization of medicine—all essential to understanding the motivations of community activists who fought for the people's control of their own healthcare. It also expands on the idea of chemical warfare—including the influence of China's experience with opium—and its pivotal role in the revolutionary use of acupuncture to combat heroin and methadone addiction.

Chapter 2 departs from the chronology to give a background on Chinese medicine and acupuncture in the United States from the early 1970s to the present, including a discussion of the scientization of acupuncture as it moved from China in the mid-twentieth century into the United States. Scientization encompassed acupuncture analgesia, which was well used as a political tool by Mao's government, and auricular acupuncture, which would become an important component of early revolutionary detox acupuncture.

Chapter 3 and Chapter 4 follow the theoretical and practical beginnings of the acupuncture detoxification program known as Lincoln Detox. The split between the (relatively) more mainstream branch of therapy, led by psychiatrist Michael Smith and leading to the development and promotion of the renowned NADA protocol for addiction, and the more politically radical branch, led by Mutulu Shakur, was a key event in the formation of revolutionary detox acupuncture. Ultimately it led to the creation of the Black Acupuncture Advisory Association of North America and the acupuncture college and clinic known as BAAANA. Chapter 3 also discusses the precarious political climate in which revolutionary acupuncture operated and the effect that climate had on efforts to establish BAAANA to serve oppressed Black and Latinx people in Harlem. Chapter 4 encompasses the lifespan of First World Acupuncture and its motivations and methods in a changed political climate. First World Acupuncture was defined by its declaration of the right of oppressed people and people of color to learn and benefit from indigenous medicine, its emphasis on serving under-resourced communities, and its struggle to sustain the vision of revolutionary acupuncture without the political engagement. It proposed a new vision for acupuncture education, presaging the existence of POCA Tech.

Chapter 5 moves into the present with a focus on POCA, the group now at the forefront of acupuncture as a sociopolitical movement. The chapter traces POCA's evolving vision as articulated by its founder, the quietly charismatic Lisa Rohleder. It also explores its potential role—outlier or influencer?—in the education and practice of twenty-first century American acupuncture.

Chapter 6 explores what became of the 1970s-era revolution and implications for the present and future of acupuncture as revolution. The chapter synthesizes the themes of scientization, suffering, and the role of love in revolutionary healing. It concludes with portraits of four contemporary acupuncturists who have been personally and professionally influenced by their knowledge of revolutionary detox acupuncture.

## Intentions

Much of the history portrayed in this book was experienced by people of color, particularly Black Americans and Puerto Ricans. There was also significant involvement of white people, some of whom were among those most dedicated to political revolution. One of the themes to emerge from the history is the division between the two branches of detox acupuncture, led respectively by the white psychiatrist Michael Smith and the Black activist Mutulu Shakur. Some of Shakur's supporters still feel bitter towards what they see as a white-coated, white-male-medical-doctor culture taking credit for a movement they started. I was asked once, while researching this book, what my intention was in writing it. It is not my intention to appropriate anyone's story. Each has their own experience; none of these experiences are mine.

My intention is to tell a history of acupuncture and revolution from multiple viewpoints to explain a world that once existed and which has had a profound but so far little explored effect on a lineage of healthcare and social justice that exists today. It is a uniquely North American history of acupuncture, while at the same time a part of Mei Zhan's "worlding" of traditional Chinese medicine. I believe the story is resonant today for multiple reasons: the increasing chasm caused by economic and social inequality in the United States and around the world; the worsening of racism and reemergence of white supremacism; the perilous terrain of our healthcare system; and the persistent faith of those who pioneered acupuncture as revolution and those who champion its use for social justice today that yes, the insertion of fine needles into people's bodies can address disharmonies both individual and social.

To my knowledge, aside from the notable exception of POCA Tech, no acupuncture college has given recognition to the revolutionary detox acupuncturists as founders of the NADA protocol, a widely used system in drug detoxification programs. Nor have they recognized the role that Black and Latinx Americans played in bringing acupuncture to underserved African American and Puerto Rican communities, while calling for healthcare as a human right. The history has likewise been little known in integrative medicine circles, which value both acupuncture and innovative access to healthcare for underserved communities. This book is intended to reach clinicians, educators, and academics in the East Asian medicine and integrative-health worlds, to give a contextualized account of this underrecognized aspect of radical healthcare history. It is also intended for practicing acupuncturists in the present and future who may take inspiration that theirs is a medicine for everyone and that its humblest use—to serve those with the fewest resources—ranks with its highest achievements.

# CHAPTER 1

# The South Bronx and Lincoln Hospital

T he South Bronx of the 1970s was an exemplar of urban decay. The reasons for the decline of the area were legion and complex. Historically, there had been successive waves of people immigrating to escape desperate circumstances; for some of these people, the South Bronx did indeed provide, for a while, a chance to live a better life. Miguel "Mickey" Melendez, in his memoir of his time as a member of the Young Lords, told of moving into an "upscale" area of the South Bronx, in the 1950s, where the neighbors were a mix of European immigrants including Catholics and Jews, which he described as the perfect neighborhood for the aspiring middle class to raise their families.[1]

By the mid-1970s, however, the middle-class dream had long since died. In its place were gutted shells of apartment buildings punctuated by rubble-strewn lots, shattered businesses, and the stench of toxic city smoke laden with the chemicals of molten infrastructure. Stretches of the Bronx could easily have been mistaken for a war zone, filled with the appalling detritus of senseless destruction. The people who hadn't left shared spaces not fit for human habitation with vermin. Families got by with no heat or hot water. Heroin addicts urinated in dark hallways.

Photographer Mel Rosenthal, who grew up in the 1940s and 50s in a solid working-class neighborhood, in what became the South Bronx, captured both the devastation and the spirit of those who remained while working for the State University of New York/Empire State College, in a building not far from his boyhood home. Shocked at what he found, Rosenthal began photographing first the devastation and later the residents of the neighborhood. Many of Rosenthal's subjects are children, their defiant playfulness juxtaposed against broken wire, garbage, or fields of unidentifiable debris. In one photo, a boy is airborne, in the midst of a front flip, over a mattress thrown across the middle of a sidewalk. Other mattresses are strewn about, their stuffing spilling out like the entrails of animals. In the background, a fire hydrant shoots water over a dented car parked in a deepening puddle littered with cans and other bits of rubbish.[2]

One of Rosenthal's students was Walter Bosque, a member of the Young Lords and a founder of what became known as the Lincoln Acupuncture Detox Collective, shortened to Lincoln Detox. Bosque recalled accompanying Rosenthal as he walked the streets looking for subjects. "You have to look at these pictures because you will not believe the conditions that people were living in," he said.[3] Conditions were still so bad in 1980 that the progressive city councilman Gilberto Gerena-Valentin appealed to the Soviet Union for foreign aid and advisers. More a publicity stunt than an expectation of change, Gerena-Valentin's plea highlighted the neglect the South Bronx was receiving from the US government.[4]

The neglect was not unintentional. In fact, a policy of "benign neglect" of struggling urban neighborhoods was proposed in January 1970 in a memo written by presidential advisor Daniel Patrick Moynihan to President Richard Nixon. The patently racist memo used data on fire alarms in New York City to suggest that many such alarms—"concentrated in slum neighborhoods, primarily black"—were due to arson caused by the inhabitants and that fires were a "'leading indicator' of social pathology for a neighborhood." The solution was to pull back fire response and other services from these neighborhoods. That policy was to have profound effects on the South Bronx, where an

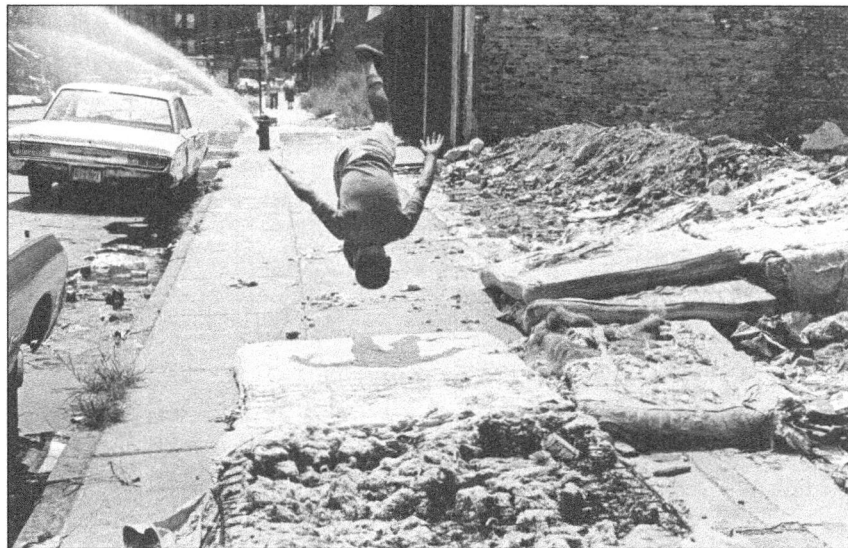

*Impromptu gymnastics on Bathgate Avenue in the 1970s South Bronx. Photo by Mel Rosenthal. Courtesy of Roberta Perrymapp and the Rubenstein Library, Duke University.*

increasing number of fires would rage out of control, displacing tenants and ultimately tearing apart communities.[5]

Benign neglect was recommended as a nationwide policy. In 1976, Roger Starr, New York City's Commissioner of Housing Preservation and Development, proposed a policy specific to the city that was also more proactive in that it would triage communities. "Planned shrinkage" would target neighborhoods essentially deemed too ill to be worthy of life support and pull the plug by cutting off municipal services. Resources could then be allocated to "healthier" areas. However, Deborah Wallace and Rodrick Wallace, who applied ecological methodology to study the relationship between fire and public health in New York City, found serious fallacies behind this rationale.[6]

Benign neglect and planned shrinkage accelerated or caused the demise of parts of the Bronx throughout the 1970s. In particular, the well-documented "burning of the Bronx" resulted in a massive loss of housing for poor people as well as white flight. Eighty percent of housing units and population in some areas between 1970 and 1980 was lost, and around 600,000 people living in poverty were uprooted by the destruction of their homes, while another 1.3 million white inhabitants fled the city for more stable areas.[7] But while the spectacular devastation led to international notoriety, it was not the first time Bronx communities had struggled for survival—or lost to forces larger than themselves.

Metaphors such as sickness, illness, decay, and death had long been employed to describe poor neighborhoods of New York, while the philosopher Marshall Berman claimed to have invented the word "urbicide," which he described as the murder of a city and used specifically to describe the South Bronx, where he grew up and from which his family was displaced.[8] Numerous social and political forces through much of the twentieth century led to urbicide in the South Bronx. There was deindustrialization, the deliberate movement of industry out of New York from 1929 to 1969, as planning decisions emphasized the use of real estate for other profit-making purposes such as finance. (Ironically, in 1969, the New York Department of Planning released its Master Plan for New York City, calling for "industry renewal" in the South Bronx and mandating that existing structures and homes be cleared to make way for new industry.) Another juggernaut was the advent of roads and automobiles as the idealized urban space. More than a way to transport those of means to the "nicer" suburbs, the emphasis on the roads themselves as the public space was a significant new phenomenon. As Berman writes of New York's master builder Robert Moses, the roads he conceived and constructed in the 1920s and 30s foreshadowed the reconstruction of the broader American landscape after World War II, in which there was a "unified flow whose lifeblood was the automobile" and cities were viewed "principally as obstructions to the flow of traffic" from which their inhabitants should be encouraged to escape.[9]

The road that wreaked the most havoc on the South Bronx was the Cross Bronx Expressway, which resulted in the demolition of 159 buildings housing 1,530 families.[10] Robert Caro devotes two chapters of his

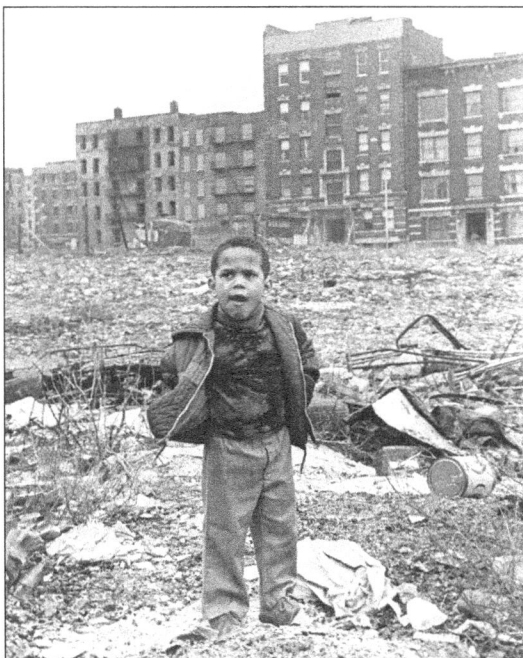

*A young boy in the South Bronx in the 1970s. Photo by Mel Rosenthal. Courtesy of Roberta Perrymapp and the Rubenstein Library, Duke University.*

monumental biography of Robert Moses to the systematic and cruel displacement of the largely working-class Jewish neighborhood of East Tremont by the road (which, as Caro describes it, could have taken a slightly different route with much less destruction).[11] Once the road was in place—a years-long process pocked by delays caused by under-budgeting—exhaust fumes from the trucks that ran past remaining city streets severely impacted air quality.[12] Families that could afford to escape did so, while poorer people—often Black or Latinx Americans—who were leaving even worse circumstances moved in to replace them.

Displacement was also caused by urban renewal policies or "slum clearing." Such policies began well before the Cross Bronx Expressway was conceived: Limits on the rights of landlords and tenants against powerful slum-clearing interests were established in the most concentrated period of the Great Reform—a time when many public health measures and workplace improvements were instituted—from 1880 to 1920. Provisions of the federal Housing Act of 1949 also greatly facilitated Moses' slum-clearing projects.[13]

Robert Moses, an unelected official but one of the most powerful figures in New York City for a good part of the twentieth century, was paradoxically famous for both his public works and his appalling disrespect for humanity. He was said to love the public but not as people.[14] He made no pretense at hiding his disdain for people; if cities had become mere obstacles to traffic, then humans were nothing more than obstacles to Moses' grandiose vision. While he had a near mythic reputation—Berman places him, at the height of his powers, in the pantheon of "titanic builders and destroyers" including Louis XIV, Joseph Stalin, and Captain Ahab—there is disagreement as to whether he was the primary agent of the changes his work wrought or a tool of larger forces. Berman thought he was both, consecutively, stating that by the 1950s Moses had fallen out of the titanic pantheon and was only fitting into a larger historical context of reconstruction and integration. Wallace and Wallace affirm that "Moses certainly didn't act in a vacuum." Yet they also credit him with, perhaps, being single-handedly responsible for New York's heroin epidemic of the 1950s and 60s.[15]

By the 1970s, even more visible than the heroin epidemic was the epidemic of fires in the South Bronx. Wallace and Wallace posit the burning of the Bronx was the key to a deliberate policy to prevent power from ending up in "hands of the wrong color."[16] They connect this policy most closely to the New York City-Rand Institute, a public/private think tank that provided data, beginning in 1969, based on severely flawed research models. Most damning is the implicit racism they claim was behind the alliance between the city and the Rand Corporation. The 1960s saw a significant shift in demographics, as millions of African Americans and Puerto Ricans moved to New York, seeking a better life. Unfortunately, their arrival coincided with the departure of the industries that had offered opportunities to previous waves of immigrants from other nations.[17] Even so, partly as a result of programs begun under Lyndon B. Johnson's War on Poverty, Black and Puerto Rican politicians, labor unions, and activists began to gain strength. Wallace and Wallace assert that the ruling powers, fearing their growing influence, combined to thwart them. Hence the relationship with the New York City-Rand Institute, and the subsequent spread of burned-out buildings and their multiple ramifications.

## Documentaries and the System

It wasn't that no one knew what was happening. To the contrary: This was the heyday of television, and the world could watch from its home while eating dinner. In 1972, an episode of the *Man Alive* documentary series, called "The Bronx is Burning," depicted the results of budget cutbacks on fire safety.[18] But the Bronx continued to burn, and five years later, a nation fixated on the second game of the World Series would witness the incineration of Public School 3, a few blocks from Yankee Stadium. Sportscaster Howard Cosell, who was covering the game for ABC, noted that President Jimmy Carter had been in the Bronx just days earlier; Carter had been personally assessing the cumulative wreckage. Some South Bronx residents recalled with dismay, however, that Cosell said the people were burning their own neighborhood rather than pointing the finger at avaricious landlords collecting insurance payouts; by this time, there was abundant evidence that some of the fires were certainly started for that reason.[19]

The year 1977 also saw the national dissemination of two critically acclaimed documentaries. The first, *The Police Tapes*, which was shown on public television, followed officers of the 44th precinct of the South Bronx as they went about their business. Much of the footage was filmed at night and has an edgy air, with crime seeming to lurk around every corner. What is most striking about *The Police Tapes*, though, is how most of the calls have more to do with social work than true crime. Officers try to persuade a middle-aged woman not to attack another middle-aged woman with a fire iron when the neighbor closes her door too loudly. They intervene when a young woman says her mentally ill older brother has taken their mother hostage in her own apartment. They talk down a group of young people from escalating a single shooting, over a minor disagreement about clothing, into a major gunfight.[20]

The second documentary, *The Fire Next Door*, focuses on the still-burning South Bronx where, in the year before the film was made, 3,500 buildings went up in flames, and between 1970 and 1975 there was an average of 33 fires each night.[21] It too tells the sorry tales of people in desperate situations. There is the elderly woman who lives by herself in an abandoned building with no heat or electricity; her only family, her three dogs, were killed when teenagers threw them off the top of the building. There is the chronically ill mother of nine, bedridden, determined to leave her son in jail in the hope he'll learn from his mistakes, at the age of 15. And there is the young mother who hasn't unpacked her furniture months after moving into an apartment because, she says, the mice will eat it. She says she can handle the sagging ceiling in the bathroom, the lack of cold running water, the unflushable toilet. What she doesn't get, she says, is why people have to throw their garbage out the window.[22]

A common thread in both films is Anthony Bouza, who serves as something of a Greek chorus to the tragedies playing out onscreen. Once the Bronx Borough Police Commander, Bouza was relieved of that position for speaking his mind, which he does logically, articulately, and with deadpan irony. (Bouza had also been one of the detectives investigating the assassination of Malcolm X in 1965 and was no supporter of Black liberation activism.)[23] Bouza compares the Bronx to Vietnam, calling both "a great moral struggle and a great moral dilemma" for Americans. He is a big-picture viewer who sees the system as the destabilizer of society. Describing the city's reaction to the increased activism, heroin addiction, and resultant methadone use of the 1960s, Bouza says, "A law enforcement administration system was created, we were showered with goodies, and now we are a very efficient army of occupation and the problem is invisible and everybody's back in business as usual and it's wonderful for everybody."[24] His assessment hits squarely on the head the issue that everyone else seems to be skirting: Who is to blame for the collapse of a society? The law enforcement answer was to round up the usual suspects. Thus, disgruntled residents looking to settle a score, punk kids with nothing but time on their hands, welfare recipients in need of a better home (who could only get one in any reasonable time if their current home burned down), profiteering landlords, and the ubiquitous junkies could all be targeted as the cause. What Bouza saw and dared to say was that it was the system driving all these individuals down their separate ruinous paths.

## Lincoln Hospital

At the beginning of the 1970s, the South Bronx had a single hospital. The Bronx and Westchester County, two of the most populous counties on the mainland of New York, rub shoulders with one another. Yet in 1969, while wealthier, and whiter, Westchester County had a hospital bed for every 93 residents, the South Bronx could offer just one hospital bed for every 4,500 residents. Westchester County boasted 28 private hospitals as well as a public one.[25] The South Bronx had only Lincoln Hospital, a public institution whose name was its most aspirational aspect: At one point in the hospital's colorful but checkered history, it had been redubbed Lincoln in an attempt to recall the spirit of its abolitionist founding. The hospital's roots took hold before the Civil War as a charitable home for elderly escaped slaves.[26] Run by the Society for the Relief of Worthy, Aged, Indigent Colored Persons—a philanthropic group chiefly made up of white women—the home moved from Manhattan's Lower West Side to the East Side, where in 1882 it became The Colored Home and Hospital.[27] In 1898 the hospital moved to newly constructed buildings at the intersection of Southern Boulevard and 141st Street in the Bronx. The move was fateful, as the population of the Bronx was mainly white at that time; soon the institution was renamed the Lincoln Hospital and Home and was opened to all races. However, the hospital did boast the only nursing school open to Black women in the United States; founded in 1898, it proved a great success in terms of expansion and career opportunities for its alumni. Nonetheless, the philanthropists had increasing difficulties raising funds and covering costs. In 1925, the hospital was sold to the City of New York Department of Public Welfare and became known simply as the Lincoln Hospital, while the nursing school was renamed the Lincoln School for Nurses. The sale marked a turning point for Lincoln. Fitzhugh Mullan, who as a radical young doctor worked at the hospital in the late 1960s and early 1970s, and who told its tale poignantly in his memoir, *White Coat, Clenched Fist*, pointed out the deficits of a welfare approach to medicine. Mullan argues that after the sale in 1925, Lincoln Hospital's finance and management were based on two simplistic principles defining welfare medicine—quarantine and protection—and that these were inadequate provisions of healthcare for poor people. Mullan's crucial point was that welfare medicine neither defines nor recognizes healthcare as a human right.[28]

By the 1950s the neighborhood and the hospital had gone through significant changes. The South Bronx was now populated mainly by Black Americans and Puerto Ricans, while the hospital had become physically outdated, poorly managed, and inadequately staffed. As it became less attractive to ambitious American medical residents and interns, an increasingly higher percentage of foreign doctors—mainly from India, Thailand, and the Philippines—filled those positions.[29] The lack of doctors who were fluent in either English or Spanish became another alienating factor for the community. Conditions in all areas deteriorated to the extent that, by 1970, Lincoln Hospital had a well-established nickname. Among Jewish immigrants fleeing oppression in Eastern Europe, Puerto Ricans looking for a way out of poverty, and African Americans seeking an escape from the violence of southern racism, it had become known as the Butcher Shop.[30]

The epithet was barely hyperbolic; healthcare in the South Bronx was truly in a parlous state. The infant mortality rate, a key indicator of public health, was 30 per 1,000 live births—double the national average. Tuberculosis infections were three times the national rate; heroin overdose was the number one cause of death among teenagers and young adults. And statistics tell only part of the tale. Rodents skittered through trash piled up in Lincoln's hallways, while levels of lead in the paint covering the walls of the pediatric wards—where children were being treated for lead poisoning—were found to be higher than in the homes those children came from.[31] Mullan depicted the hospital's condition as an outdated, cockroach-infested war zone. He described it as lacking in every key area, to the extent it became essentially a triage station.[32] Indeed, much of Lincoln's business constituted emergency care; its emergency room was ranked the busiest in New York and the fourth busiest in the United States, although the hospital's 346-bed capacity was just a fraction of that of many other urban public hospitals.[33]

## The Affiliation Program and Medical Empires

Community unrest had been brewing for years at Lincoln before Mullan's arrival. The first takeover of one of the hospital's programs was in 1969, and it stemmed from a rising discontent caused by what was known as the Affiliation Program. The plan, launched in 1961, invited private hospitals and medical schools to partner with the city's struggling public hospitals, recreating the latter as teaching institutions. Each of New York's 21 municipal hospitals would be managed by one of the state's private medical schools or centers. The idea was that the private institutions, contracted to supply high-quality staff and professional direction, would raise the standards of their poorer partners to an equivalent level. In practice the program was riddled with flaws and bitterly disputed by the municipal hospitals' constituents.

The Affiliation Program was perhaps fatally flawed from the start, conceived by the "medical-industrial complex" to create "medical empires" at a time when awareness of, and intolerance for, imperialism was becoming a central part of healthcare activism. The terms were coined by the Health Policy Advisory Center (Health/PAC), an independent think tank that had a close relationship with New York healthcare activists beginning in 1967. Under the medical empire interpretation, Lincoln's patients were "teaching material" for the upper-middle-class medical residents and interns from the wealthy and paternalistic Albert Einstein College of Medicine, its affiliation partner. The term was understood to denote Black and brown patients; white patients, in contrast, were understood to be customers. Lincoln Hospital was thus seen as a colonial outpost serving as a training ground for Einstein's medical residents and interns.[34]

Unlike the American Medical Association (AMA), which had fought bitterly against Medicare, stakeholders in the so-called Einstein-Montefiore empire, which encompassed Lincoln, were liberal medical reformists. But they were also elite, white, and part of the medical-industrial complex that fed the research-and-development appetite of the capitalist machine. They concentrated intellect, finances, and power at their centers, while expanding into ghettoes for their own enrichment. They determined relationships with banks, construction firms, real estate agents, insurance companies, and drug and hospital supply chains, further embedding municipal healthcare into the existing power structure. They monopolized public funds for health education and research, neither of which provided much direct benefit to the health needs of the community; indeed, health research sometimes led to unnecessary and harmful diagnostic or therapeutic procedures. And their physical expansion had destroyed neighborhoods and uprooted local health facilities.[35]

The central truth to the Affiliation Program was an imbalance of power. The author and activist Barbara Ehrenreich wrote later of her time at Health/PAC,

And our job … was not to tell the people what to do, or what to ask for, but to tell them where to go, to tell them where to find the power. That was the point of all our research on the medical empires and medical-industrial complex and all the huge structures of government agencies that had been set up: to locate power, so people could see how to go after it.[36]

Health/PAC wrote of the "hegemony" of the medical schools and their philanthropic partners, who were given quotidian operating powers of the city's entire hospital system and generous subsidies to run it. Over 25 percent of the city's municipal hospital budget was spent on Affiliation contracts. In 1969, Einstein received $7.5 million (approximately $54 million in 2020 dollars) for its affiliation with Lincoln. Yet, as Ehrenreich wrote in 1970, "Lincoln Hospital is owned by the City, staffed with professionals by Einstein, and neglected by both."[37] A report from the Institute for Policy Studies in 1967 was sharply critical of the program, revealing that benefits to patients were not nearly as substantial as advertised.[38] There were also accusations of financial mismanagement and fraud; investigations in 1967 and 1968 found evidence that Affiliation contracts had been used for purposes ranging from payroll-padding to outright fraud, while a 1969 inquiry discovered that Einstein had used Affiliation money for new and unrelated equipment and jobs, leaving its programs at Lincoln severely understaffed.[39]

The last point in particular led to the dismay, disgust, and finally fury behind the takeover of Lincoln's community mental health services program in the first week of March 1969, which Health/PAC described as "one of the year's most militant, and least publicized, labor actions."[40] Einstein had launched numerous programs at the hospital with its Affiliation budget, but the community soon perceived these as a sham. A key part of the program was to train community health workers to staff mental health clinics housed in walk-in storefronts. A brief but poignant documentary—later used by the Health Revolutionary Unity Movement (HRUM) to energize further action at Lincoln—recorded the environment before, during, and after the takeover. "It quickly became clear it was just a paper plan and we were window dressing for Einstein's liberal reputation," said one worker in the film. The walk-in clinics were underfunded, understaffed, and overwhelmed with need. Wait lists were so long that eventually the young women answering the endlessly ringing phones began turning everyone away. If patients were allowed in, it was only long enough to fill out a couple of perfunctory forms, and then they were told to seek help elsewhere. Clinic workers tried making house calls, but there was no budget for cars or taxis, and public transit was so slow that one call could take half a day. The clinics' daytime schedule was inaccessible to many working people. Because human resources were so inadequate, treatment consisted mainly of drugs, an especially galling outcome, as the community was acutely aware of its street drug problem and activists were promulgating the message that the system was pushing street drugs to keep the people down. Morale was so low that one clinic worker said, "Even if we could have operated an evening clinic, it would have meant bad health care 24 hours a day instead of the usual eight."[41]

On March 4, 1969, around 150 community clinic workers took control of Lincoln's mental health services. The immediate catalyst for the action was the firing of four employees, but workers said the discontent had been brewing for the four years the program had been running. Instead of shutting the program down, however, employees continued to run it in some capacity, with support from the community and some professional staff, for weeks. The action was pointed directly at Einstein: We the people will not abandon our own, no matter how bad the conditions you leave us. The workers' demands seemed simple enough: better services and better control of community services. After all, the most publicized part of the mental health services was the storefront clinics dotted around the area, staffed in large part by the specially trained community employees. But tension over the right of the community to control its healthcare remained at the crux of all the disputes, including more comprehensive hospital takeovers, to come. This tension was central to the struggle to introduce a drug detoxification program at Lincoln and later to bring acupuncture training and treatment into the South Bronx and Harlem.

The background to the mental health services takeover is significant to an understanding of the later events at Lincoln, which led to the development of the acupuncture collective. First, some of the activist mental health workers would become members of two collectives, the Think Lincoln Committee and HRUM, which were among the influential groups to force changes at Lincoln in the early 1970s. Second, some key theoretical underpinnings of the 1969 takeover presaged the context in which future actions would occur.

## Professionalism

One such theme involved the fraught distinction between professionals and paraprofessionals or nonprofessionals. For community employees of the mental health services program, the point was laden with connotations—first of all, race. Nearly all the paraprofessional workers were Black or Puerto Rican, while the professionals were white. Secondly, it highlighted the stranglehold on upward mobility the professional class exerted on other workers. For instance, Einstein hired unemployed or underemployed South Bronx residents as part of a "new careers" program meant to educate and train community mental health workers and set them on a path for career progression. However, a top position for such paraprofessionals, that of community organizer, was restricted to college graduates. Some of the workers were given the opportunity to study for a degree, but they came to see the offer as a move to pacify the more militant staff. Others who received some formal education found it was neither relevant to their jobs nor led to commensurate pay raises or promotion.[42] Finally, for some activists who were studying the writings of Mao Zedong and Che Guevara, the division of workers into professional and other groups was a central flaw of capitalist society.

Professionalization quickly became a critical issue for community activists who learned acupuncture. Acupuncture could not legally be practiced without a license and, in the 1970s, licenses were mainly restricted to medical doctors. New York's first law regulating acupuncture was passed in 1974 and required the license holder to already have a license outside of New York and to have practiced acupuncture for at least 10 years. Medical doctors, though, could take a 50-hour course and gain a license. In truth most New York acupuncturists were Chinese and practiced outside the law; they would have been considered nonprofessionals, while an MD could take in a brief overview of acupuncture technique and practice legally as both a professional acupuncturist and a doctor.

The professional/nonprofessional or paraprofessional duality was also relevant to the barefoot doctor program. A key feature of the barefoot doctor program was that it bypassed the need for professionalism by training young peasants to use both indigenous medicine and simple Western medicine techniques for many common conditions. The barefoot doctors brought previously unavailable basic treatment to their own communities. The concept appealed to young, radical medical students and doctors, who were drawn to the idea of using simpler, more natural techniques employing commonly available resources. They were also impressed with the use of indigenous medicine, which appealed to their countercultural sensibilities.[43]

Training volunteers as nonprofessional acupuncturists was thought of by the early members of the Lincoln acupuncture collective as a way of bringing a simple, natural treatment from the people to the people. However, they were mainly successful in doing this outside the law. Passage of another law in 1992, which grants a license to acupuncturists who have undergone formal training and passed exams, tightened regulations still further. Sonia Lopez, a medical doctor who worked with acupuncturists at Lincoln in the late 1970s, said, "Some of the acupuncturists who had been barefoot doctors couldn't pass the exam." She was referring not to Chinese medics but to acupuncturists trained by the collective at Lincoln, showing, again, the degree to which the barefoot doctor concept had been absorbed. Lopez added, "I'm learning how these things calcify things and exclude people."[44]

Another theory underlying the 1969 takeover was that health can only be understood in the context of social factors. Social systems can make a person sick; to be healed, the person's relationship to society must change. In a practical sense, changing a person's relationship to society might mean changing their living situation. One of the mental health services employees described a typical scenario: "If the man was depressed and he lived in a rat hole, we went out and helped him, and we carried his bed on our backs. In other cases we started putting pressure on the landlords." To the workers' consternation, if not surprise, the system prevailed: "Then word came down from the man: 'We don't move patients anymore, cool it.' We found out later that one of the landlords was a big contributor to Einstein."[45]

By this analysis, the client's depression stemmed from having no choice but to live in a rat hole. A necessary part of the healing process was getting him a better place to live. The understanding that health is a holistic matter, and that environmental, physical, and mental health are intertwined, fit with traditional Chinese medicine theory. The practical lifestyle help given the man also embodied the spirit of the barefoot doctors. One US newspaper article, from 1968, described how a young barefoot doctor climbed a tall hill every day to look after a 70-year-old woman who lived alone and was paralyzed. The article noted, in a sarcastic tone, that the young man was praised by Chinese authorities for doing the woman's laundry and for manifesting "true love of the people."[46] His actions would have seemed natural and praiseworthy to the community activists of the South Bronx; members of the Lincoln acupuncture collective and its offshoots were clear, in my conversations with them, in maintaining they were acting out of love for the people.[47]

The understanding of health as a function of social determinants went much deeper than the importance of individual living situations, though. Intimately bound up with the problem of healthcare in the South Bronx was that of drug addiction, and those activists who began focusing on it believed the only way to dig out the root of addiction was to rid society of poverty, racism, and sexism—and the resultant exploitation and alienation of entire classes of people—through socialist revolution. In their determination to revolutionize healthcare was an explicit criticism of the capitalist system as the source of social ills and individual illness alike. Thus, the fight to heal individuals was also a battle cry against capitalism and another facet of Third World Marxism's anticolonialism. Alternative modes of healing were seen in themselves as remediation against the destructive forces of a capitalist society—a tool of revolution.

# "Welcome to the People's Hospital"

The Black and Puerto Rican community mental health workers who orchestrated the 1969 Lincoln mental health services takeover, with support from white professionals, had been assisted in their negotiations by an assortment of community representatives, ranging from clergy to the BPP. The Black Panthers, however, were not formally part of subsequent actions at Lincoln. Three movement groups coalesced to tackle Lincoln head on: the Young Lords, Think Lincoln, and HRUM. The Young Lords focused their actions on improving health in the community. Think Lincoln emerged in the spring of 1970—a mix of Puerto Rican and white, nonprofessional and professional, hospital workers allied with community activists (including street gangs). Its sole purpose was to improve conditions at Lincoln. HRUM, an organization of hospital workers, was formed in opposition to the labor unions at another New York municipal hospital, Gouverneur Hospital in Manhattan's Lower East Side, in the fall of 1969. By the end of that year, HRUM had become allied with the Young Lords, and its work began spreading to other public hospitals. Like several of its contemporary movements, HRUM published a multipointed plan and a newspaper. The plan focused on community health, community control, and workers' control; the newspaper, *For the People's Health*, was aimed at educating the community and spreading the movement to other hospitals. HRUM formed a Lincoln Hospital chapter following the community mental health services takeover and subsequently took on a primary role in directing actions there.[48]

Mullan believed the most notable of HRUM's 10 points was its first: a demand for community-worker control of all health services in the communities. The distinction of community-worker control (versus community control), wherein workers are brought in as key actors because they have a degree of ownership of their workplace, was new and important, Mullan contended. Indeed, it was the worker part of the equation that would become paramount: By 1972, Health/PAC claimed the slogan "community-worker control" was shifting towards "worker control." It was the hospital workers—who spent much of their lives in the hospital and understood its mechanisms—who had forced the small but significant changes at Lincoln. Members of the community, in contrast, were less familiar with the hospital's workings, tended to use it only in times of personal stress, and were more physically disparate, making coordination less likely.[49]

On June 17, 1970, Think Lincoln proffered a list of seven demands to Dr. Antero LaCot, Lincoln's new administrator. (LaCot, a Puerto Rican gynecologist, had been appointed in February at the insistence of Lincoln's Community Advisory Board.) Demand number four took center stage as the activists requested an immediate decision on their request for a round-the-clock grievance table for patients and workers alike. LaCot hesitated, and the next day Think Lincoln set up a table in the lobby of the emergency room. It was soon flooded with complaints. The activists—lacking formal power to address them—used direct action where possible; for example, in response to complaints of long wait times, they tracked down doctors taking long lunch breaks and told them to return to work. The doctors reportedly corrected their behavior.[50]

A march and rally were subsequently held, at the end of June, by Think Lincoln and the Young Lords to demand action and community control of the hospital. The march was marred by police violence; 10 marchers were arrested, and reportedly beaten afterwards, including three who were "seriously beaten and tortured" at the police station.[51] The rallies were followed, on July 14, by a smoothly executed takeover of the old nurses' residence, where residents and interns grabbed an hour or so of sleep when they could. The activists made their move before dawn but planned for the eventuality of hand-to-hand combat with police, arming themselves with weapons of Asian combat, nunchakus and shurikens, or throwing stars.[52] The occupiers had also planned for publicity, alerting the media to a press conference soon after securing their stations and raising a Puerto Rican flag. Bilingual banners made of sheets were flown from the windows, declaring, "Bienvenidos al Hospital del Pueblo" and "Welcome to the People's Hospital." A day of press attention and negotiations, primarily with the somewhat sympathetic Lacot, ensued, surrounded by heavy police presence.

The medical staff, like everyone else at Lincoln, was taken by surprise. Yet a significant portion of them supported the takeover. Mullan and other young medics formed another group of activists dedicated to transforming Lincoln. These doctors had belonged to the Student Health Organization (SHO), the radical organization for medical students rebelling against the complacency and elitism of the AMA and its student offshoot, the Student American Medical Association. While it lasted only from around 1965 to 1970, SHO had a lasting effect on many doctors who came of age during the period. Mullan had helped form what was known as the Lincoln Collective, a group of medical doctors and residents who had belonged to SHO. The collective's aim was to effect change in the medical system—and by extension practices at Lincoln—from within, and they assisted or joined, to various degrees, radical groups working outside of Lincoln for similar purposes.[53] While there was a constant tension between the dominant paradigm—i.e., white doctors from the medical establishment—and the people's or "Third World" movements comprised mainly of Black and Puerto Rican community members, many of the actions at Lincoln, and such changes as occurred, could not have been achieved without the collective's participation.

Lincoln was quite an attraction to radical young doctors. Some came from Albert Einstein College of Medicine, Lincoln's affiliation partner; others came from Columbia University's medical school. Columbia was contracted to manage Harlem Hospital, but Lincoln's "butcher shop" reputation exerted a magnetic effect on doctors who had spent their student years as activists. These doctors formed the Lincoln Collective. While they did not formally join with any of the community activist groups—they were most closely allied with an offshoot of HRUM, the Health Revolutionary Alliance, from 1971 to 1972—they did provide practical training to activists and financial support, for instance, to print newspapers or as bail for jailed movement members.[54] And in actions at the hospital, although they were frequently not involved in the planning and found themselves playing catch up, their support was important and perhaps crucial at times. For instance, late in the day of the takeover on July 14, 1970, the occupiers left the building quietly and without violence or arrests. The situation could have been much different. As Mullan describes in *White Coat, Clenched Fist*, members of the Lincoln Collective met with the Young Lords and devised a plan whereby the doctors would accompany the occupiers, a few at a time, through the heavily armed ranks of police. The police swore at them as they passed but could do little else.[55] Other activists left surreptitiously through windows. The role of the doctors was not reported in the memoir of Young Lords leader Mickey Melendez, *We Took the Streets*. By Melendez's account, over 100 activists just disappeared, despite the heavy police presence.[56] A report the next day by New York's *Daily News* stated only, "The police, who entered the building at 5:40 p.m. through a first-floor window when they found the front door locked, conducted a floor-to-floor search which revealed that all the militants had left."[57] On the other hand, Mutulu Shakur specifically gave credit to "doctors who put their lives and careers on the line" during and after the takeover.[58]

The July takeover of the nurses' residence was a symbolic victory for the activists. However, substantive change remained elusive, and conflict continued to percolate. It erupted again just two weeks after the occupation, following the death of a young Puerto Rican woman named Carmen Rodriguez after an abortion performed at the hospital. Rodriguez, a mother of two, had been in a residential drug treatment program outside of Lincoln but had been diagnosed at the hospital with rheumatic heart disease, where doctors discovered her pregnancy and recommended an abortion. Doctors who reviewed her chart did not dispute the recommendation but were outraged by the decision to use a saline infusion, a highly risky procedure for someone with heart disease.[59] The event led to another round of demands from the Young Lords and Think Lincoln, with support from the doctors of the Lincoln Collective, ultimately triggering both the departure of the head of Obstetrics and Gynecology and an injunction from the newly formed

Health and Hospitals Corporation against anyone "interfering with patient care and medical services" at the hospital.[60]

The tragic death of Carmen Rodriguez also marked a milestone bold step by one young physician. Dr. Michael Smith, a resident in psychiatry, had been working with the drug program Rodriguez had attended. Smith accessed her hospital medical chart and, accompanied by citizen representatives from the complaints table, entered the administrator's office and reported the controversial contents.[61] It was Smith's action—judged valiant by some, reckless or even illegal by others—that precipitated the outcry over her death. Smith was to become an important figure in Lincoln's acupuncture detoxification program, but some revolutionary detox acupuncturists ultimately came to view him as representing the establishment he worked for. In 1970, though, he was nearly discredited by that same establishment for his courageous action in support of the South Bronx community.

The events surrounding Rodriguez's death illustrated, even more starkly, the extent to which the doctors of the Lincoln Collective were woven into the fabric of the radical political movements operating in the hospital. They not only provided support to the activists but initiated and participated in actions against the hospital's establishment. There was a schism between the collective doctors and the generally older, more established doctors, some of whom called for criminal action against Smith. So strong was the difference in feeling that, while the collective doctors occupied the office of the head of the Health and Hospitals Corporation to demand change, the entirety of the obstetrics staff walked out in support of their director and remained on strike for 10 days. Only after Einstein was threatened with the loss of its contract to manage Lincoln under the Affiliation Program were the striking doctors persuaded to relent.[62] Nonetheless, the college's dean, Dr. Labe Scheinberg, and Dr. Elmer Foster, the hospital's chief of radiology and president of its medical board, agreed that, in the months after Carmen Rodriguez's death, the hospital was under de facto control of the medical doctors' collective. This internal support was critical to the footholds established by the community activists.

The broader social establishment was more grudging than the hospital administration in admitting any ground had been ceded. While Joseph T. English, head of the Health and Hospitals Corporation, allowed he was "encouraged by the fact that new talent is being attracted to the hospital, talent that may be better equipped to handle the problems of the 70s than some of the older doctors who may have battle fatigue,"[63] the New York Times editorial board saw things differently. "A potentially historic experiment … to see whether ghetto hospitals could be used to radicalize poor Blacks and Puerto Ricans much as leftist students have used the universities to radicalize other student and faculty … has not gone well for the radical cause," opined an editorial dated September 6, 1970. The piece claimed the Young Lords had "important allies within the hospital, a group of radical young physicians … Some of these are revolutionaries dedicated to destroying 'oppressive capitalism.'" The editorial concluded that the Young Lords and the community had lost credibility in trying to force changes as a result of their actions after Rodriguez's death.[64]

Notwithstanding that opinion, activist groups were, if anything, emboldened. Another amalgam of activists engineered a second occupation of the hospital in November 1970, this time demanding a drug treatment program. At the time, Lincoln offered nothing more than emergency care for acute drug use complications and nothing at all to remediate chronic drug abuse. The groups involved included Think Lincoln, HRUM, the Young Lords, and a significant number of present or former drug addicts. Dr. Franklin Apfel, a member of the doctors' collective and later medical director of Lincoln's acupuncture detoxification program, recalled they were "mainly made up of ex-addicts who had been in prison for some ten to fifteen years and were politicized—Muslim, Black Liberation and Puerto Rican nationalists—and wanted to do good for the community."[65] The takeover, of the sixth floor of the house-staff administration building, was once again supported by doctors from the collective, who gave the occupiers keys to their on-call rooms on the sixth floor. The area was swiftly transformed into an ad hoc detoxification unit, with several of the occupiers started on methadone. The organizers issued their demand: a 100-bed detoxification unit to be controlled by community members, including those struggling with addiction. However, under authority of the recent injunction, 15 people were arrested, and the activists were removed by police on the same day.[66] While it was short-lived, the action had an enduring response: In January 1971, the state awarded a seven-figure grant to fund a drug detoxification program at Lincoln.[67] It was this program that evolved into the Lincoln Acupuncture Detox Collective.

## Chemical Warfare

The second occupation of Lincoln Hospital, and its aftermath, have been viewed through various historical lenses; in Melendez's memoir, they were a natural follow-up to the July action led by the Young Lords; to many involved in acupuncture detox today, the second takeover has been conflated with the first to form a singular defining event that occurred at Lincoln Hospital. What has been overlooked is the tremendous importance of the concept of "chemical warfare" to the development of acupuncture as a revolutionary means of addressing addiction, illness, and social inequity.

The analysis of chemical warfare began with a growing consciousness of a web of global sociopolitical relationships involving international drug trade and heroin addiction, particularly of Black and Latinx Americans and Vietnam veterans. Such relationships were described in pamphlets disseminated among activists, which highlighted the relationship between colonialism and the opium trade. In 1972, the US historian Alfred W. McCoy's *The Politics of Heroin in Southeast Asia* was published, detailing the role of the CIA and other US government agencies in perpetuating heroin trade and addiction through its actions in Southeast Asia during the Vietnam War. The book laid out a scenario in which the American government's anti-Communist zeal trumped all other concerns.

The CIA became the vanguard of America's anti-Communist crusade, and it dispatched small numbers of well-financed agents to every corner of the globe to mold local political situations in a fashion compatible with American interests. Practicing a ruthless form of clandestine realpolitik, its agents made alliances with any local group willing and able to stem the flow of "Communist aggression." Although these alliances represent only a small fraction of CIA postwar operations, they have nevertheless had a profound impact on the international heroin trade.[68]

Specifically, McCoy writes,

During the early 1950s the CIA had backed the formation of a Nationalist Chinese guerrilla army in Burma, which still controls almost a third of the world's illicit opium supply, and in Laos the CIA created a Meo mercenary army whose commander manufactured heroin for sale to American GIs in South Vietnam. The State Department provided unconditional support for corrupt governments openly engaged in the drug traffic. In late 1969 new heroin laboratories sprang up in the tri-border area where Burma, Thailand, and Laos converge, and unprecedented quantities of heroin started flooding into the United States. Fueled by these seemingly limitless supplies of heroin, America's total number of addicts skyrocketed.[69]

Although McCoy describes these actions as an "inadvertent but inevitable consequence of … cold war tactics" he contends the United States was actively and knowingly engaged in illegal heroin trafficking:

American diplomats and secret agents have been involved in the narcotics traffic at three levels: (1) coincidental complicity by allying with groups actively engaged in the drug traffic; (2)

abetting the traffic by covering up for known heroin traffickers and condoning their involvement; (3) and active engagement in the transport of opium and heroin. It is ironic, to say the least, that America's plague is of its own making.[70]

McCoy's work was, predictably, contested by the CIA. Before its publication he was called, on June 2, 1972, to testify before the Foreign Operations Subcommittee of the Senate Appropriations Committee. McCoy, at the time a doctoral student at Yale, was questioned about his claims that "the CIA provided substantial military support to 'right wing rebels, and tribal warlords who are actively engaged in the narcotics traffic,'" and that "in Northern Laos, Air America aircraft and helicopters chartered by the US Central Intelligence Agency and USAID [United States Agency for International Development] have been transporting opium harvested by the agency's tribal mercenaries." Following his testimony, McCoy spoke to reporters, to whom he elaborated on the use of Air America's aircraft to transport opium for the Meo tribesman of Laos.[71] While McCoy's testimony was sharply disputed by some members of Congress—notably Senator Gale W. McGee (D-Wyoming), who accused the academic of engaging in McCarthyism—his work has been well received in academia. Hardly a fringe figure, McCoy now holds an endowed chair at the University of Wisconsin; the third edition of his book was published in 2003, with the more direct title *The Politics of Heroin: CIA Complicity in the Global Drug Trade*.

Even before the publication of McCoy's book, leftist thinkers and the Black Power movement had linked heroin to the pacification of ghetto inhabitants, suggesting it was used by institutionalized powers to thwart their capacity to engage in revolution. Such powers were seen through the lens of anticolonialism and anticapitalism that was pervasive among New Left and liberation movements. The Young Lords picked up the message and purveyed it, for instance, with a graphically worded article in the first edition of their newspaper, *Palante*.[72] Other activists also began speculating that the CIA played a role in perpetuating heroin addiction on US streets. Angela Davis later spoke of it, describing drug abuse as responsible for the pacification of revolutionaries and militants.[73]

The allegation has never been proven. Deborah and Rodrick Wallace, in *A Plague on Your Houses*, correlate drug overdoses to the burning of the Bronx; neighborhoods that received influxes of refugees from the resulting destruction saw increases in overdose figures. They relate the behavior to post-traumatic stress disorder similar to that suffered by Vietnam War veterans as well as to the loss of communities, which may have been poor but still provided stability.[74] Nonetheless, it was with the belief in federal government involvement that Mutulu Shakur would flesh out his interpretation of chemical warfare while developing revolutionary detox acupuncture. Chemical warfare provided the background to Shakur's revolutionary approach to acupuncture. Barbara Zeller, who was involved in both revolutionary detox acupuncture and First World Acupuncture, provided insight into his analysis: "The movements themselves were becoming flooded with heroin. [That affected] the number of people that could get organized into resistance. People were getting strung out, and their [the activists'] position was drugs were not being stopped coming into the community. They knew of the relationships with the CIA bringing in drugs and the Golden Triangle."[75] Zeller's comment adds nuance to the activists' stance: She references McCoy's findings, but in noting "drugs were not being stopped" she pulls up short of claiming the government was deliberately pushing heroin on the streets. Still, the anticapitalist, anticolonialist understanding of the heroin trade and addiction laid the ground for the detoxification movement.

## Addiction and Methadone Maintenance

The problem of heroin addiction in the early 1970s was immense. Addiction was prevalent in urban areas across the United States but nowhere more so than in the Bronx.[76] In addition, to the dismay and shock of their families, a significant proportion of young men returning from Vietnam were addicted to heroin. The solutions offered by society, however, were as problematic as addiction itself. Society treated addiction as a matter of personal responsibility and failure; clean up the individual, and the problem goes away. Thus, drug use and possession were crimes punishable by the state, whereby drug users were put away, out of sight of society. The criminal approach was intensified by President Richard Nixon, who in 1970 signed into law the Controlled Substances Act, which classified drugs according to their medical usefulness and potential for abuse. Nixon tightened the reins even further when he launched the "War on Drugs" in 1971. The "war" led to changes, notably increasing federal funding for drug-control agencies and mandatory prison sentencing for drug crimes, whose impact resonates today.

Beyond imprisonment, there were detoxification programs meant to wean addicted people off heroin. The most popular method, known as methadone maintenance, was developed and promoted by physicians at Rockefeller University, a prestigious private establishment in Manhattan that boasted the oldest biomedical research institute in the United States. The Rockefeller family had long been involved in foreign medical and scientific research institutions; in China, its PUMC was the most influential training center for physicians in the early part of the twentieth century. (In a presumably deliberate twist of irony, the college was renamed the Anti-Imperialist Hospital during the Cultural Revolution.)[77] Under methadone maintenance, methadone—like heroin, an opioid-class drug—essentially replaced heroin as the drug of addiction. One might fairly ask what the difference was between addiction to one opioid or another. While methadone had been used effectively in acute situations to reduce the severe symptoms of heroin withdrawal, the main difference between the two was that methadone was legal while heroin was not. Both drugs led to addiction, withdrawal from either caused severe side effects, and both resulted in thousands of overdose deaths. Indeed, in Washington, DC, outside the Capitol building and the White House where government legislators sat, the number of deaths from methadone overdoses surpassed that for heroin in 1971. Yet methadone maintenance was given broad-scale approval by the Food and Drug Administration (FDA) in 1972, despite an alarming amount of evidence of the potential dangers of the drug and of the inadequacies of maintenance as a detoxification system.[78]

Perhaps the greatest drawback of methadone maintenance was that it perpetuated opioid addiction in such a way that the user was reliant not on street dealers but on the government for the next fix. Such dependence left users at the whim of state dictates. For instance, parole status and the receipt of welfare benefits depended on adherence to the program, and permission to be in the program could depend on whether the user conformed to social norms of hairstyle or dress. There were also political repercussions. People reported being harassed or threatened with expulsion from their programs for wearing political buttons supporting Black liberation movements.[79] Michael Tabor, a member of the Black Panthers, claimed that methadone was used as leverage to get addicts to act as spies by reporting on revolutionary talk in the streets.[80] There were also reports of people being arrested on showing up for their methadone dose, allegedly after the police tracked their schedule through government-controlled clinic records.[81] Finally, the state not only acknowledged but condoned methadone addiction as a means of control. Dr. Peter Bourne, an influential figure in methadone maintenance, wrote in a manual for the Department of Justice and the Law Enforcement Assistance Administration:

> At the center, the patient is exposed to all of its rehabilitation services, including his relation with his counselor … which can evolve into one of trust and intimacy with considerable therapeutic potential. The fact that methadone is addictive is essential to allow this to occur. Many addicts have difficulty establishing close relationships and were it not for the fact that they were addicted, they would find it extremely difficult, if not impossible, to return reliably on a daily basis and establish an ongoing relationship with the personnel of the clinic.[82]

The history of methadone itself gave still more cause for suspicion of a state promoting its use. Michael Smith, who as a psychiatric resident had led activists in protesting Carmen Rodriguez's death, gave testimony at congressional hearings on the heroin epidemic in 1976, which he later adapted for the radical magazine *Science for the People*. As Smith explained, by 1972, the pharmaceutical giant Eli Lilly was responsible for 90 percent of the methadone used both legally and illegally. Lilly had been a mainstay in keeping heroin in medicine cabinets, namely as cough medicines, after the 1914 Heroin Narcotics Act banned most narcotic drugs in the United States. After World War II, Lilly joined with the State Department in an investigation of Nazi drug companies; one of the drugs that had been developed in Germany during the war was an opioid narcotic called Adolphene, in honor of Adolph Hitler. Within two years Lilly was marketing a cough medicine called Dolophine, the active ingredient of which was Adolphene, now known as methadone.[83] The connection of a "therapeutic" opioid narcotic to the Fascist perpetrators of the Holocaust resonated with the experience that Black Americans had with the medical establishment, as articulated by Mutulu Shakur: "The disrespect, the indifference and the failure to provide information necessary to make meaningful decisions is associated with the historical arrogance of the status of 'white coats' in treating us as guinea pigs for their drugs, therapies, research and experiments."[84]

The history of opium use was equally fraught with connotations of abusive medical and political powers. Opium had been used medically since ancient times and into the nineteenth century when it was commonly included in popular pharmacy medications in England. Opium led to morphine and then to heroin; each were regarded, in their time, as wondrous cures with the ability to "kill all pain and anger and bring relief to every sorrow."[85] Each was developed as a substitute for the one before it, as each one was found to be dangerously addictive—just as methadone would be in the twentieth century.

Morphine was synthesized from opium in 1805 and developed as an injectable drug about 50 years later. During this time it became a clinically valuable anesthetic; however, it soon proved to be as addictive as opium. The search for a nonaddictive painkiller led to heroin, synthesized in 1874 by English researcher C. R. Wright under the chemical name diacetylmorphine. Within 20 years, German scientists were hailing it as an effective treatment for common respiratory illnesses and as a nonaddictive substitute for morphine and codeine. The German company Bayer first manufactured the new drug as heroin and in 1898 launched an international advertising campaign.[86] Heroin was approved for general use by the AMA, and recommended in place of morphine for infections, in 1906. But in less than two decades it became evident the new drug caused the same old problems of addiction; in 1924, the deputy police commissioner of New York City reported that 94 percent of drug addicts arrested for crimes were heroin users. In the same year, Congress unanimously voted to ban the import or manufacture of heroin.[87] Internationally, the Geneva Convention of 1925 strictly regulated the manufacture and export of heroin, and the Limitation Convention of 1931 stated heroin's manufacture must be limited to medical and scientific needs. While these measures reduced the legal supply of heroin, illegal production and trade increased.

The role of colonialism in narcotics addiction was detailed in a thoroughly researched booklet called *The Opium Trail: Heroin and Imperialism*, which was authored collectively by a study group "with support from the Committee of Concerned Asian Scholars."[88] *The Opium Trail* was circulated among activists concerned with drug addiction in the 1970s and became a central text for students at the acupuncture college established by Shakur, under the auspices of BAAANA. The booklet describes a centuries-long trail of colonialism and addiction leading from British and American empire building and trade dominance in India and China to the contemporary Vietnam War. It lays out a compelling case, depicting the opium trade as the key to financing the colonialists' expansion and power, including Japan's role in China during World War II. That history is linked to the war in Vietnam—along the lines of McCoy's thesis—through the US government's role in propping up the corrupt elite of Southeast Asia, who receive military weapons, financial aid, and a tacit wink as they profit from illegal heroin trade, the text argues. Moreover, the United States supplies a vulnerable population of potential consumers in its military forces, who fall prey to heroin in their need to escape the reality of war. The narrative turns full circle as the same power structure, in its perpetuation of an inherently unjust social system, creates the need for addiction and feeds that addiction on the streets of American cities.

China's experience with opium addiction is emphasized for two reasons: China suffered particularly from the opium trade; and it made an extraordinary recovery from opium addiction after the Communist takeover in 1949. The emphasis on China was important to the development of the detox program at Lincoln. China was held as a model for eliminating addiction because it addressed the root of the problem, i.e., that society, not individual weakness or pathology, was to blame for drug abuse. Only radical social change, on both a societal and an individual level, could reverse the epidemic. The emphasis on social change as a necessary precursor to individual healing was also resonant with the community workers' approach in the Einstein/Lincoln mental health program.

China's solution was described as twofold: first, getting rid of profiteers, whether foreign or local; second, rehabilitation of individuals through political education. When drug abusers were able to see themselves as victims of a corrupt old order while envisioning a new society full of opportunities for them, they would be able to recover. There were pragmatic measures too, notably detox programs providing free drugs under an accelerated withdrawal schedule and job opportunities with related education.[89] The principles of political education and accelerated withdrawal were to become cornerstones of the first detox program established at Lincoln following the November 1970 occupation. Almost certainly the China model was an inspiration; Melendez, in *We Took the Streets*, said that the Young Lords studied the experience of Mao's China in combating opium addiction.[90]

The Young Lords were also influenced by the writings of Michael Tabor and Joshua S. Horn. Tabor, a BPP member who had battled heroin addiction, been held in prison as one of the Panther 21, and self-exiled to Algeria during the subsequent trial, left behind a pamphlet called *The Plague: Capitalism + Dope Equals Genocide*, which followed a similar line of argument to *The Opium Trail*, although written in more graphic language. (Tabor was quoted in the front of *The Opium Trail*, where he was described as "Michael Tabor, ex-junkie, now a black revolutionary.")[91] Horn was a British physician who, in the mid-1950s, moved to China for self-described political reasons. His memoir, *Away with All Pests: An English Surgeon in People's China: 1954-1969*, is an account of his experience in its medical system, including the use of acupuncture and the nascent barefoot doctor program.[92] Horn's memoir (named after a line in a poem by Mao Zedong) makes clear his full-scale approval of Mao's revolution as the cause of a drastic improvement of healthcare in China. He also lauds the emphasis on rural and peasant healthcare, which he links to a need for radical healthcare reform where other Third World revolutions were taking place in Asia, Africa, and Latin America. Horn argues that China not only made much-needed improvements to its healthcare system but that, in uniting the traditional and the modern through collective action, it surpassed the standard of medical care in Western countries.

Along with the pervasive media attention given the barefoot doctors, Horn's book, published in 1969, likely influenced activists with its message of the success of collective community action in revolutionizing healthcare. Horn also describes accurately and succinctly the basic theories of traditional Chinese medicine as well as how it was incorporated into Chinese hospitals. He depicts how traditional bone setting was combined with modern methods as an example of the success of this approach but only briefly mentions the use of acupuncture. Interestingly, Melendez recalled that Horn's memoir described the role of acupuncture in "great detail" for various conditions, including drug rehabilitation.[93] As Horn does not mention drug rehabilitation, the idea of using acupuncture for detox must have come from another source.

Thus, among revolutionary activists, there was a coming together of the ideas of socialism, China, and acupuncture as healing forces in opposition to the destructive historical powers of capitalism, imperialist

Western governments, and state-sanctioned pharmaceutical therapy—or abuse. Mao's teachings and the principles of Third World Marxism, as discussed in the previous chapter, provided a theoretical basis for the idea that East Asian modes of healing could be used to combat a perceived state of war involving heroin/methadone addiction. This blend provided fertile ground for the detoxification program that took root at Lincoln in the early 1970s. Within a few years, it bloomed into the controversial but highly successful acupuncture detox program—a program that would form, and be informed by, revolutionary detox acupuncture. The following chapter will explore acupuncture's transition during the latter part of the twentieth century from a largely esoteric practice to a modern form of medicine. In particular, the chapter will examine the "scientization" of acupuncture beginning in Mao's era and the effect of that process on contemporary American acupuncture.

CHAPTER 2

# The Long Project
# of Scientization

A North American who wants to try acupuncture in the second decade of the twenty-first century has a panoply of options. In the United States, acupuncturists may be available in holistic health spas, doctors' clinics, integrative cancer-treatment centers, and individual offices. There are acupuncture franchises as well as shop-corner-style practices. You can get a community treatment in a room filled with reclining chairs or a one-hour personalized session in a private room. The patient may pay a set fee, a figure based on a sliding scale, or a copayment through an insurance plan. Beginning with the passage of the Patient Protection and Affordable Care Act in 2010, insurance coverage for acupuncture was expanded in some regions; in California, for instance, the state with by far the highest number of licensed acupuncturists in the country, acupuncture was designated an "essential health benefit" as of 2014, meaning it would be covered by both federally subsidized plans and unsubsidized plans for some conditions.[1]

Despite these advances, access is not universal or equally distributed. Studies of acupuncture use have shown that patients tend to be white, female, middle-aged, in the middle-to-upper income brackets and relatively well educated.[2] While Medicaid, the federal and state insurance program for certain low-income and vulnerable groups, may cover acupuncture in some states, the reimbursement rates are often so low that acupuncturists will not accept them. Historically Medicare, which provides health insurance to nearly one in five Americans, has not paid for acupuncture for any condition. In 2020, the law was changed to allow acupuncture treatments for chronic low back pain only, with a maximum of 20 visits annually.[3]

Acupuncturists are not equally distributed across the United States. Nearly one-third of licensed acupuncturists in the United States practices in California, 12 percent in New York, and 7 percent in Florida—comprising over half of the national total. Per capita, the states with the highest numbers are Hawaii, Oregon, and Vermont, closely followed by California and New Mexico.[4] Even within these states, licensees are spread unevenly; New York City, not surprisingly, has the highest number of New York acupuncturists, while the Bay Area, Los Angeles, and San Diego County account for a majority of California practitioners. The distribution is in part due to the location of acupuncture colleges, which are also heavily concentrated in California, Florida, and New York. (The East and West coasts together house more than three-quarters of US acupuncture colleges.[5]) The uneven allocation may also correlate with levels of income, which, as noted above, tend to be higher in those who utilize acupuncture.

Acupuncture education is not uniform, but a strong degree of conformity is required for colleges to meet the standards of the Accreditation Commission for Acupuncture and Oriental Medicine (ACAOM), the national accrediting body. The standards are based on knowledge of TCM, the brand of Chinese medicine developed under Mao's government beginning in 1956. Students quickly learn to note the irony that a system called "traditional" eliminated many branches and aspects of the indigenous medicine; however, these have not all died out but are now more properly referred to as "classical Chinese medicine." Some colleges offer education outside the TCM paradigm; for instance, the College of Classical Chinese Medicine at the National University of Natural Medicine in Portland, Oregon, and the Jung Tao School of Classical Chinese Medicine in Sugar Grove, North Carolina.

Whether classical Chinese medicine or TCM, acupuncture degree programs usually take four years to complete and include theoretical and practical training along with clinical internship. Colleges have their own clinics, which charge reduced prices to clients and are generally quite popular in the neighborhoods they serve. Most offer additional clinical training at offsite locations, ranging from programs for underserved populations such as those suffering from drug addiction, homelessness, or domestic abuse to integrative services in high-profile hospital systems. The nonhospital offsites also provide a valuable service to the community, bringing free healthcare to people who are medically and financially vulnerable. Somewhat like the barefoot doctors, modern American acupuncturists receive some training in biomedicine as well, including anatomy, pathophysiology, physical exam, and differential diagnosis, and are taught to recognize red flags and when to refer patients out.

Once students graduate, they must pass board exams before they can be licensed. Licensure falls under state jurisdiction, and indeed not all states have laws regulating acupuncturists, although the number is diminishingly small; only Alabama, Oklahoma, and South Dakota remain unregulated.[6] Most states require graduates of accredited colleges (who receive a master's degree in Chinese medicine or "Oriental medicine") to pass some or all of the four National Certification Commission for Acupuncture and Oriental Medicine (NCCAOM) exams to acquire a license. The exams cover foundations of "Oriental medicine," acupuncture and point location, Chinese herbology, and biomedicine. Depending on which exams are passed, the graduate will receive certification in "Oriental medicine," acupuncture, or Chinese herbology, and in some states only an acupuncture certification is required.

An acupuncturist's professional title also varies by state. As discussed in the introduction, professionalism can be a contentious issue for healthcare providers. Not least among these are licensed acupuncturists, who have waged a long campaign to be recognized by the conventional healthcare system. Most licensed practitioners want professional status within the system, and to this end acupuncture colleges have recently developed an academic path leading to the title "Doctor" for the majority of graduates.

Why does it all matter? First, there is historic precedent for the battle for respect from the biomedical community. A century ago, traditional medicine practitioners in China were threatened with career extinction as biomedicine proponents began a campaign of complete domination of the medical field. While the comparison is inexact on many counts, the diminution of a potent traditional medicine by the controlling biomedical paradigm today still threatens both practitioners and patients—the former in terms of their ability to earn a living, the latter in terms of their healthcare choices and ultimately their health. Second, acupuncture is a vital part of the integrative health movement. There is no conclusive definition of the concept of integrative health, but it includes the understanding that healthcare is a matter of cultivating health at least as much as treating illness and that lifestyle and various nonconventional approaches can be combined with conventional medical care for optimal results. Integrative health is not a new concept, but it is an evolving one. To date, it has not evolved sufficiently to move beyond the domination of biomedicine; thus, acupuncturists are trying to integrate on biomedical terms, including the professional status of "doctor."

It will take more than nomenclature to make the necessary shift for acupuncturists to be considered equal partners in healthcare. An example is the recent Medicare legislation allowing payment for acupuncture for chronic low back pain. Under the law, medical doctors can administer acupuncture with no additional requirements, and physician assistants and nurse practitioners/clinical nurse specialists may do so if they have an acupuncture degree from an accredited school and a valid acupuncture license. Licensed acupuncturists, qualified as "auxiliary personnel," are only allowed to perform acupuncture for Medicare reimbursement under supervision by an individual in one of the above categories.[7]

This cumbersome situation, which arises more from the way the status quo is embedded in bureaucracy than from a deliberate attempt to marginalize acupuncturists, raises the matter of professional competition.[8] Medical doctors can practice acupuncture with relatively few hours of training or none at all, depending on the state, compared to the minimum 2,625-3,000 hours of clinical and academic training required for a licensed acupuncturist.[9] In some states, chiropractors, dentists, nurses, osteopaths, physician assistants, and physical therapists can also practice acupuncture with minimal or unspecified training.[10] The acupuncture treatments they give are technically called "medical acupuncture" (in the case of those with a medical license who have received specialized training) or "dry needling" (in the case of physiotherapists or chiropractors). Such therapy may bypass the traditional diagnostic techniques and underlying theories of Chinese medicine. The basis of medical acupuncture or dry needling simply becomes anatomy or point function. An example of the former would be needling a point called Neiguan (Pericardium 6) on the distal inner aspect of the forearm to treat carpal tunnel syndrome, based on its proximity to the median nerve; an example of the latter would be using the same point to relieve postsurgical or chemotherapy-induced nausea. While there is no scientific research to date definitively explaining the antiemetic mechanism of Neiguan, its classical indication for that purpose is backed up by extensive clinical effectiveness research.[11]

The plethora of clinical research evidence for certain common conditions treated by acupuncture has eased the way for practitioners with a firmer hold in the conventional healthcare system to use acupuncture in a limited fashion. The problem for licensed acupuncturists is that the conventional healthcare system does not recognize its use of acupuncture as limited. The subtle arts of pulse-taking, tongue examination, questioning, and palpation; the critical aspect of pattern diagnosis; and the range of modalities including moxibustion, tui na massage, and herbal formulas are lost in the more mechanistic approaches of medical acupuncture and dry needling.

Even for acupuncturists who limit themselves to acupuncture, there are many different systems and microsystems that can be employed when simple point functions or anatomy are not enough or to hasten the effect of treatment.[12] Moreover, Chinese medicine can effectively treat a far wider variety of conditions than are currently condoned by health insurers, who purportedly base their decisions on the results of clinical research. It might appear, then, that scientific research has done a disservice to licensed acupuncturists. It delineates the conditions they can be reimbursed for treating, while encouraging physicians, chiropractors, and others to use acupuncture without comprehensive Chinese medical training. Yet scientific studies have been extremely important for the acceptance and development of acupuncture in the United States and elsewhere.

## The Scientization of Acupuncture

The project of "scientizing Chinese medicine" was a vital feature in the development of modern Chinese medicine under China's Nationalist government (1928-1949). The medical historian Sean Lei, in *Neither Donkey Nor Horse*, his masterful analysis of the modernization of Chinese medicine, points out that "scientize" (*kexuehua*)—a commonly used word in China, Japan, and Korea today—has no counterpart in the Western world, although the concept of science originated in Europe.[13] Perhaps the implication is that the Western world can conceive of nothing outside of science, whereas in East Asian countries, the imagination retains a capacity for other natural systems. Of course, there was no need for the word in China before the advent of science and no need to apply it to Chinese medicine until the latter was under threat from biomedicine.

Lei dates the appearance of the slogan "scientizing Chinese medicine" to somewhere between 1915 and 1925 but states it did not become popular until the early 1930s with the creation of China's Institute of

National Medicine ("national medicine" being the name traditional practitioners chose for their medicine, tying it to the power of the state in their struggle to keep it alive and relevant). The meaning of "scientize Chinese medicine" was not entirely clear at the start; however, a central tenet that Lei repeatedly emphasizes is that science and traditional Chinese medicine do not have to be antithetical. Although the historical background is entirely different, I would argue that the spirit of the project—that Chinese medicine can exist in the modern world only after being transformed into a medicine compatible with science—was transplanted onto American soil with acupuncture's arrival in the United States.[14]

Just as physicians and academics were intrigued by their glimpses of the barefoot doctors, so were many of them fascinated by the practice of acupuncture—particularly acupuncture anesthesia during surgery. Both phenomena were heavily advertised and promoted by the Chinese government as astonishing evidence of what the Communist revolution had produced. Both certainly lent themselves well to the purpose, as eye-catching uses of indigenous traditions adapted to the modern world. Coincidentally, just as China was modernizing, many in the West—particularly young people—were seeking out natural alternatives to modern conveniences and to esoteric practices and beliefs in place of Anglo-European ways. Indeed, acupuncture was latched onto not only by the revolutionary activists in New York but contemporaneously by a small contingent in the psychology department at the University of California, Los Angeles. This group, which anthropologist Tyler Phan calls the "UCLA cohort," became highly influential in establishing some of the first acupuncture colleges in the United States and, perhaps more importantly, in professionalizing acupuncture through the passage of acupuncture laws.[15]

In California, acupuncture gained a strong following after it was legalized in 1975. The state began regulating acupuncture in 1972, but from 1972 to 1975 the practice was controlled by the Board of Medical Examiners and authorized only under supervision of a licensed physician for the purpose of research in medical schools.[16] This stipulation would seem to force the "scientization" of acupuncture as soon as it rose into the popular view. In fact, that appears to have been the intention of the UCLA cohort. Phan quotes William Prensky, one of the cohort members, as saying that in contrast to chiropractors, who had established themselves outside of medicine and lacked privileges and recognition from the medical community, "We had a different political idea, which was to move into the middle of medicine and set up a tent."[17] The regulation did benefit mainly the UCLA cohort, and Phan argues the issue was one of power between a dominant and a marginalized group. Implicit in that relationship is that the culture of science (a group of psychology researchers) was attempting to seize control of a traditional healing practice. In doing so, the researchers would tame its enigmatic reputation through scientific analysis.

## Acupuncture Anesthesia

Other physicians and researchers were also very curious about acupuncture, due in no small part to China's promotion of acupuncture anesthesia. They were particularly attracted by the use of an electrical current running through the needles, called electroacupuncture, frequently used during surgical procedures to enhance the needling effect. In 1973, C. Norman Shealy, a neurosurgeon who had been investigating modes of electrostimulation to reduce pain, suggested the reason Americans suddenly became interested in acupuncture was the addition of electricity. "Electronics and electricity offer some semblance to known science," he wrote in a paper exploring the mechanisms of electroacupuncture. "Thus, the incorporation of electrical current into acupuncture allows the Western mind to think seriously about it without having to acknowledge embarrassment at the previously expressed ignorance and even indifference."[18] Medical anthropologist Elisabeth Hsu also emphasizes the scientific import of acupuncture anesthesia in impressing both the Chinese and the West. Noting that acupuncture analgesia (pain relief through needling) had existed for centuries, she questions why it became a heralded phenomenon seemingly overnight at the

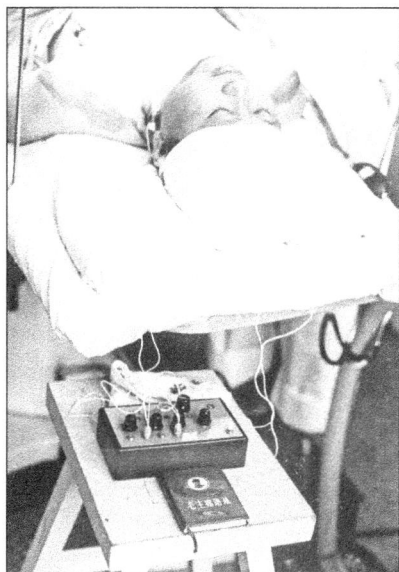

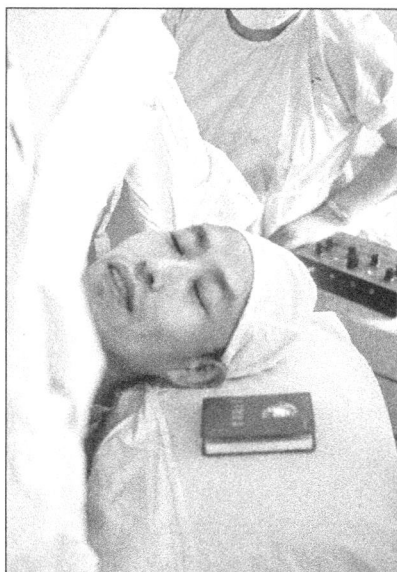

*Patients undergoing surgery using electroacupuncture at Beijing Medical College in 1971. Left, a copy of Mao's quotations is touching the electrostimulation machine, attached via wires to the acupuncture needles. Right, an electroacupuncture machine is visible in the background. Patients were said to prepare for surgery by attending Mao Zedong Thought classes. Photos by Paul Pickowicz. Courtesy of Paul Pickowicz and University of California San Diego Library.*

end of the 1950s. (Shortly after the first known surgery using the technique was reported, 47 more procedures were performed in less than three weeks in Shanghai, while it simultaneously appeared in two other regions.) Hsu's answer is that, "The proof that acumoxa [denoting the related techniques of acupuncture and moxibustion] had physiological effects was now given, the results could be seen; acupuncture analgesia provided the evidence that Chinese medicine was a science."[19]

However, the value of acupuncture anesthesia to the Chinese government was only one part science. It was at least as much a demonstration of political devotion to Mao. Paul Pickowicz, who as a young

PhD student involved in the Committee of Concerned Asian Scholars was among the first American academics to tour modern China (in 1971, the year before Nixon's groundbreaking visit), took scores of photos on his journey. His group was invited to observe four surgeries using acupuncture anesthesia; his photographs show a little red volume of Mao's quotations placed carefully next to the patient's head in one case, while in another *The Little Red Book* is touching the electroacupuncture machine. Pickowicz found the surgeries disconcerting but was impressed at the apparent lack of pain the patients evinced (of a woman having a cataract removed, he said her anxiety and discomfort seemed "nothing at all like the pain I was experiencing as a witness").[20] After the surgery he describes the woman announcing, "Chairman Mao has given me back my sight." When the scholars asked how surgical candidates prepared for the ordeal, they were told that patients participated in "Mao Zedong Thought" classes.[21]

Pickowicz mentions another aspect to the politics of acupuncture anesthesia. His group's hosts, he said, wanted them to witness "self-reliance" via a scientific development. Paul Unschuld gives the concept a more thorough treatment in his monumental analysis, *Medicine in China: A History of Ideas*, relating the use of acupuncture anesthesia to the effort to establish dialectical materialism as a core principle of modern Chinese medicine. He quotes Mao: "Dialectical materialism … holds that external causes are the condition of change and internal causes are the basis of change."[22] This belief, Unschuld contends, easily incorporates the classical Chinese understanding of disease etiology, whereby an imbalance of "correct" internal influences allows "evil" external influences to penetrate, resulting in illness. As he points out, acupuncture, and particularly acupuncture anesthesia, create a unique opportunity to use a purely external stimulus—one which employs no drugs and leaves the patient in an alert, active state—to engender an internal will in the organism to transform itself back to a healthy state.[23]

Enthusiasm for acupuncture anesthesia waned after the 1970s when it was still heavily promoted for ideological reasons. Unschuld's book includes a translated text from a group of physicians who claim to have conducted more than 30,000 surgeries under acupuncture anesthesia from 1969 to 1977, which they say was 1.5 percent of the national total. The physicians tell a sobering tale of patients pressured to withstand severe pain without showing a reaction; they even report that "some resorted to shouting political slogans during surgery."[24] In other cases, they say, patients were injected with anesthetic drugs sufficient to relieve pain, and then needles were inserted in their ears to give the impression of acupuncture anesthesia, after which the patients gave glowing reports of the experience. The physicians assert the technique should only be used in the patient's and surgeon's best interests, implying that had not been the case, and that it should not be enforced through administrative policies. Ironically, given this was a procedure presented to, and perceived by, the West as a great scientific advancement, they admit to "entirely neglect[ing] the procedures and methods of scientific research" in widely expanding its use.[25] Ultimately, the surgeons suggest that acupuncture anesthesia may fall out of practice entirely. As Hsu observed, that was the case by the late 1980s.

Acupuncture anesthesia, clearly, was not a pure example of "scientization." And yet acupuncture did become highly scientized (indeed, the primary legacy of acupuncture anesthesia is research into pain).[26] How did acupuncture—which had fallen out of favor for nearly two centuries leading up to, and including, Republican China—become so popular in the middle of the twentieth century, and why has it been the subject of so much scientific study?

## Acupuncture's Reemergence

Lei states that acupuncture became marginalized in Chinese medicine during the Late Imperial period, as people "increasingly abhorred the idea of intrusive intervention."[27] While that encompasses a broad time span, he narrows it when citing a renowned physician, Xu Lingtai, who, in the mid-eighteenth century, sought a teacher of acupuncture but could not find one. Hsu references the sinologists Gwei-Djen Lu and Joseph Needham in noting that acupuncture was abolished in China in

1822 "for reasons of 'injuring propriety and refinement.'"[28] Certainly by the beginning of the era of modern Chinese medicine, which Lei places in the 1920s, acupuncture was not considered significant. That attitude began to shift as a result of the continual exchange of ideas between Japan and China regarding traditional medicine, despite political conflicts between the two countries. Japan had, during the Meiji era, effectively shut down the practice of herbal medicine but had continued licensing practitioners of acupuncture and moxibustion. Lei posits it was the influence of Japan that led the creators of China's Institute of National Medicine, in the early 1930s, to include these modalities (which both fall under the scope of "acupuncture" today) as one of four major areas of reform.[29] However, if there is one personage who effected the modernization of acupuncture, it was Cheng Dan'an (1899-1957), credited by the medical historian Bridie Andrews as "the moving force behind rehabilitating acupuncture and transforming it into elite, learned Chinese medicine."[30]

Cheng was trained in both Chinese medicine and biomedicine. He reportedly became enamored of acupuncture after his father, also a physician, treated his recalcitrant back problem with acupuncture (perhaps the most common way that Americans today are introduced to acupuncture). Cheng was influential in a number of ways: He founded the Society for Research into Chinese Acupuncture, the first such institution in the country, which also incorporated the first school of acupuncture in modern China; he wrote the school's textbooks, among them the seminal *Chinese Acupuncture and Moxibustion Therapeutics*; and he redefined acupuncture points by using Western anatomy to locate them. Notably Cheng's points avoided major blood vessels, which Andrews sees as a major shift from the earlier practice of bloodletting. In contrast to the theory of releasing blood to remove blocks and induce smooth flow, Cheng explained needling action in terms of nerve stimulation. He further refined treatments by advocating the use of filiform needles rather than the thick, rough needles of the past and of using moxibustion to warm rather than blister the skin. Andrews affirms "there is no doubt that Cheng was successful in his attempts to make acupuncture scientific."[31]

From a contemporary perspective in which evidence-based medicine is the rule, the scientization of acupuncture makes sense; indeed, it is necessary for acceptance in a world in which insurance companies, medical doctors, and healthcare systems must be convinced there is some objective evidence to support its use. Proponents of acupuncture and integrative medicine have contributed hundreds of research studies to the scientific literature over the last few decades. Among the most productive clinical researchers are those looking at the benefits of acupuncture for cancer patients, an integrative approach known as oncology acupuncture that began roughly 20 years ago.[32] Prior to that, basic science researchers were already investigating the mechanisms of acupuncture.

Yet research has not been definitive. Many clinical studies have been small due to lack of funding or have lacked some feature of rigor in design. For acupuncture to be more widely reimbursed by healthcare systems—whether for cancer patients, insurance plan members, or underserved populations—further well-designed, large-scale clinical trials will be called for. But what is a well-designed acupuncture study? The answer continues to evolve based on what has been learned in the last half-century of research, not only about acupuncture but about how best to conduct clinical studies of complex whole-systems interventions. The following section gives a more detailed background of the path acupuncture research has traveled and where it stands today.

## Acupuncture Research

Quantitative acupuncture research asks three broad questions: Does it work, how well does it work, and how does it work? The first is a question of efficacy (is it more effective than a placebo under controlled conditions?), the second of effectiveness (does it compare favorably to usual care or another therapy under real-world conditions?), and the third of mechanism (what changes take place on a physiological level that indicate it has an effect?). The first two questions can be answered through clinical research, while the third requires a basic science approach.

The multiple approaches raise a chicken-and-egg conundrum. Which came first: interest in the mechanism or interest in the clinical efficacy/effectiveness? The answer is not entirely clear; however, from a scientific point of view, the question of how something works is often paramount. Among the first modern researchers to seek answers to how acupuncture works was Ji-Sheng Han, who began his basic acupuncture studies in 1965. Much of Han's prolific research used rabbits or rodents and measured the levels of various chemicals such as neurotransmitters in response to acupuncture or electroacupuncture. Among Han's significant findings, supported independently by the work of Bruce Pomeranz of the University of Toronto, was that acupuncture analgesia is mediated by the release of endogenous opioids.[33] Han and Pomeranz also found, separately, that different frequencies of electrical stimulation result in the release of different chemical mediators, and that while either low- or high-frequency electroacupuncture has an analgesic effect, the effect takes place along different pathways depending on the frequency.[34] Subsequent to Han's earliest studies, other basic science researchers examined the mechanisms of electroacupuncture in particular; electrical stimulation tends to be used more in research than it is clinically, in part because it is easier to quantify than manual stimulation.

While the basic scientists were establishing biological plausibility in animals, clinicians in the West were still wondering if acupuncture works in humans and, if so, how well. For the increasing number of patients in Europe and the United States, clinical evidence may have been beside the point; what mattered was how they felt after a treatment. But for acupuncture to gain the medical recognition the UCLA cohort craved, and to be made more widely available to all, the conventional healthcare system required scientific evidence of its efficacy. That meant randomized placebo-controlled trials, the so-called gold standard of research—widely implemented at the behest of the FDA, which in 1962 began requiring that new drugs be proven effective through controlled clinical trials before they could be approved. The move marked a significant shift from the previous policy under which manufacturers needed only to demonstrate safety.

Acupuncture clinical research proliferated in China, Europe, and the United States. Much of the research from China, though, was either not translated into English or not accepted by the Western research establishment as meeting the highest scientific standards. Some of the discomfort from the West regarding Chinese studies has to do with their frequent use of Chinese medical terminology, which is based on a different paradigm than that of biomedicine. The complaints about scientific standards are partly due to methodology; Chinese researchers were late to adopt the randomized controlled model, and many studies have been conducted with no control group at all.[35] Lack of a control group results in a high risk of bias in a study's results. There is also suspicion of publication bias, a phenomenon whereby studies with positive results are published, while those with negative results are not. Publication bias is not unique to China; however, it seems likely there has been more interest in promoting positive results of acupuncture in China than in the West, where neither the government nor many researchers have had a strong interest in acupuncture's success. A notable point of difference between Chinese and Western studies, which may affect results, is the typical "dosage" of acupuncture in China; treatments are far more frequent, often daily for two weeks, apart from weekends. Furthermore, the needling itself is stronger and more aggressive. Western acupuncture, whether in a clinical or research setting, tends to be given once or at most twice weekly, and neither the acupuncturists nor the patients want pain involved.[36]

In the West there has been significant international collaboration within the relatively small clinical acupuncture research community. From the mid-1990s to the early 2000s, several trials took place in Germany, the United Kingdom, and the United States that would prove influential among clinicians, researchers, policymakers, and payers.[37] The studies looked at various pain conditions, including chronic low back pain, neck pain, shoulder pain, osteoarthritis of the knee, and migraine and tension headaches. While acupuncturist and researcher

Steven Birch argues the studies from Germany were seriously flawed by trying to answer both sociopolitical and academic questions at once, the results were largely positive for acupuncture.[38] Most notably, the German Federal Joint Committee of Physicians and Health Insurance Plans, analogous to the National Institutes of Health (NIH) in the United States, used the results of a large German study on chronic low back pain as the decisive factor in naming acupuncture an insured benefit for the condition.[39]

## The Placebo Effect

That study (referred to as GERAC for "German Acupuncture Trials") had a perplexing outcome for acupuncturists, however. It involved three comparison groups: one received real, or verum, acupuncture; one received placebo, or sham, acupuncture; and one undertook "conventional therapy," a nonprotocol combination of drugs, exercise, and physical therapy that varied considerably among patients. The results showed that both verum and sham acupuncture significantly improved low back pain, and both significantly outperformed conventional care. The perplexing part was that verum acupuncture (using real needles inserted with stimulation at typical depths in traditionally defined acupuncture points determined by an expert panel) did not seem to work any better than sham. The latter used real needles, but the insertion was shallow, there was no stimulation, and any "known" points or meridians were avoided. As the correct choice of points and needling technique are considered very important in achieving outcomes, the results threw practitioners into a quandary. The researchers themselves questioned the underlying mechanism of acupuncture and asked whether it was even necessary to learn the traditional acupuncture points.[40]

Some acupuncturists, Birch among them, question the epistemological founding of the study, as it was conducted in Germany, where only MDs perform acupuncture. As German doctors usually have substantially less training than licensed acupuncturists, doubt was cast on the quality of acupuncture administered in the trial. However, numerous other studies conducted outside of Germany using sham controls found similar results: Both sham and verum acupuncture work better than usual care, but verum does not have a significantly greater effect than sham.[41] Since sham is meant to represent a placebo, the implications were fairly devastating. It seemed the sometimes-miraculous, pain-relieving effects of acupuncture might be due, primarily if not entirely, to the placebo effect.[42]

Another large back-pain study in the United States added yet more consternation. Sponsored by the NIH through the National Center for Complementary and Alternative Medicine (NCCAM),[43] it was intended to show definitively that acupuncture's effects were above and beyond placebo. The results, described by Ted Kaptchuk as a "disaster," indicated quite the opposite.[44] The study design ultimately included four arms: individualized verum acupuncture based on TCM diagnosis using points that varied by patient; standardized verum acupuncture using one set of predefined points; sham acupuncture using toothpicks to stimulate the points used in the standardized group; and usual care. After eight weeks of treatment, the individualized, standardized, and sham groups all displayed significantly more improvement in function and symptoms than the usual care group. And, as in the GERAC trial, there was little difference among treatment groups, including the patients stimulated with toothpicks. Once again, a prominent study's authors were left questioning the purported mechanisms of acupuncture and raising the possibility it could all be due to the placebo effect.[45]

As it happened, by the time the study took place, Ted Kaptchuk had become deeply involved in placebo research at Harvard Medical School. His studies have brought enormous insight into placebo as a genuine healing component of all types of medicine. Some of his best-known results come from studies of patients diagnosed with irritable bowel syndrome (IBS). One study, for example, found that placebo effects can be separated into components—assessment/observation, a clinical ritual, and supportive patient/practitioner interaction—that can be combined to produce incremental improvement in IBS symptoms.[46] Another showed that IBS patients in an open-label trial, who were given pills clearly identified as placebos that contained no medicine, had significantly more improvement in their symptoms than patients not given the pills. The key difference appeared to be that the active group was told that placebo is known to have powerful mind-body healing effects.[47]

Kaptchuk's work has illuminated the vast potential of placebo, yet he believes there is much more to acupuncture than the placebo effect. He attributed the bemusing results of the NIH study to a design quirk; all patients in the study, he said, were given a TCM diagnosis before treatment, a ritualistic form of attention that his own work suggests would magnify the effect of any therapy.[48] The research community's relentless focus on the needles alone had caused it to miss the more important components of a treatment, Kaptchuk and others had come to believe.[49]

There is another important feature of clinical trial design that some researchers believe has obscured the difference between sham and verum acupuncture: trial size. Large numbers of participants are needed in order to detect small but clinically meaningful differences between groups. The measure of the difference is called the effect size, often classified as small, moderate, or large. Observed effect sizes from acupuncture studies show the difference between verum acupuncture and usual care is moderate, while the difference between verum and sham is small. Hugh MacPherson, a leading acupuncture researcher from the UK until his death in 2020, and others from the Acupuncture Triallists Collaboration, determined that in order to detect the observed difference between verum and sham acupuncture, a two-arm trial would need a study sample of more than 1,000 participants—far larger than most acupuncture studies.[50] It may be that most of the clinical acupuncture trials were simply underpowered to detect these small but meaningful differences. Combining and reanalyzing the results of several high-quality studies such that nearly 18,000 patients from the United States, the United Kingdom, Germany, Spain, and Sweden were included, the Acupuncture Triallists Collaboration found statistically significant differences between verum and sham acupuncture across all the pain conditions studied: chronic headache, neck and back pain, osteoarthritis, and shoulder pain.[51]

The results represented an important step: A group including some of the highest-powered acupuncture researchers in the United States and Europe, and funded in large part by the NIH, had shown definitive evidence that acupuncture was more than a placebo.[52] More recently, over the past two decades, research using functional magnetic resonance imaging has demonstrated that blood flow to certain cortices of the brain is increased by acupuncture needling and that the use of real acupuncture has a different effect than the use of sham. In a paper published in 2017, a team at Massachusetts General Hospital, led by neuroscientist and acupuncturist Vitaly Napadow, showed that real acupuncture needling in patients with carpal tunnel syndrome produced changes in the brain that corresponded to measurable improvements in wrist nerve function. Moreover, those brain changes were associated with long-term symptom improvement. Sham needling, in contrast, produced only subjective symptom improvement.[53] Their results indicate that real needling not only has a significant clinical effect above and beyond sham but that it acts via a different mechanism than sham.

## Qualitative Research

At this point it would appear that acupuncture has been fully scientized in the Western world. Yet many of the scientists themselves have become dissatisfied with this process over the last two decades. They agree with Kaptchuk that something essential about acupuncture has not been captured by sham-controlled research. Especially in the last 10 years, with support from the burgeoning integrative health movement, acupuncture research has focused increasingly on effectiveness research, asking how well it works compared to usual care alone, other modalities, or as an adjunct to conventional medical care. The focus has been particularly welcomed by integrative oncologists and oncology patients as they seek ways to mitigate the deleterious effects of cancer treatment—in other words, ways to feel better. "Feeling better" can be hard to quantify, but it is a key component of the acupuncture experience that can encompass mood lift, improved energy, motivation, relaxation, and calmness. Qualitative researchers were asking questions such as, "Why do people initiate or continue acupuncture treatment?" or "What does someone experience while having an acupuncture treatment?"—all the while the debate over sham, mechanisms, and the placebo effect played on.

One of the earliest, ground-breaking studies to incorporate qualitative methods sought to find who used acupuncture in the United States and why they valued it. C. M. Cassidy distributed written surveys to acupuncture patients in five states. Her results were published in two parts, with Part I establishing the demographics of the study sample. Despite the range of states, the cohort was not notably diverse—nearly 90 percent white and almost three-quarters female, mainly aged 30 to 60, well educated and professionally employed—which was consistent with populations from earlier research. Part I also gave the results of questions as to what extent and in what ways participants believed their health and quality of life had changed through acupuncture. More than 90 percent said their complaints had "disappeared" or "improved," while a majority reported improved quality of life and the use of fewer prescription drugs and doctor visits.[54]

The qualitative analysis, published in Part II, found that participants valued what Cassidy called "expanded effects of care," which were "improvements in physiological and psychosocial adaptivity."[55] The former included reduced reliance on drugs, less of a tendency to experience side effects of medication, and quicker recovery from minor infections and surgery. Examples of the latter were increased self-awareness; a feeling of being centered, in balance, or whole; and the introduction of significant life changes. (Both these realms of experience provide insight into how acupuncture treatment can benefit people addicted to drugs.) The study also evoked themes of a close patient-practitioner relationship and a sense that acupuncture treats the whole person or is holistic. Cassidy defined holism as a philosophy and a theoretical model for healthcare, including five features: that health is a positive state; that it resides in the mind, emotion, spirit, and social body as well as the physical body; the idea of individual responsibility for health; the importance of health education; and the priority of gentle, natural, or low-tech interventions. Notably, Cassidy's holistic healthcare model looks much like that adopted by the revolutionary acupuncturists in New York, although they added political education as well.

Later studies, several of them in the UK, supported Cassidy's results, and continued to develop the concept of holism in acupuncture. Charlotte Paterson and Nicky Britten found participants described both "symptom effects" and "whole-person effects."[56] They identified two categories for whole-person effects, "changes in energy and strength" and "changes in personal and social identity," which they equated with Cassidy's "improvements in physiological coping" and "improvements in psychosocial coping." The authors concluded that while the components were distinct, they were indivisible and "linked together into a holistic whole."[57]

In a later study Paterson and Britten looked at how acupuncture delivered in different settings affected the experience of holism. They found that patients treated with traditional acupuncture had the most holistic experience as they had multiple problems and general health treated at once. These patients also described developing a new understanding of how to relate to their own bodies. "Western-style" or medical acupuncture, on the other hand, rarely evoked references to holism as the treatment tended to focus on a single symptom. The third setting was acupuncture given in a clinical trial. Here holism was found to be largely absent as patients were treated for one condition only, with limited practitioner/patient communication.[58] The researchers concluded: "Our research suggests that holism—being treated as a whole person— is most important to patients with complex problems, especially where there is co-morbidity and emotional upset."[59] This qualitative finding offers another insight into how acupuncture can help people who are marginalized, oppressed, suffering from trauma, or struggling with addiction.

Qualitative acupuncture research is a paradox. It seeks in a sense to "unscientize" the scientization of Chinese medicine by using scientific methods. It is inconceivable that acupuncture could have gained a foothold in the Western world without being subjected to the scientific method, and much has been learned from quantitative research about the mechanisms and actions of needling. Qualitative research has also contributed valuable insights about the psychosocial effects of acupuncture treatment. "Acupuncture treatment" implies more than mere needling and can result in subtle effects in mood and energy as well as personal change over time. Yet, despite the knowledge gained from science, most acupuncturists and even some patients place great value on retaining the spirit of the indigenous medicine as known through its theories, ancient texts, and legends. Indeed, some would argue these comprise part of the therapeutic ritual of Chinese medicine.[60]

## Auricular Acupuncture

Needling itself is remarkably adaptable to theoretical variation. If we consider that some kind of physiological change takes place with the insertion of a needle—and research since Han's and Pomeranz's work on endogenous opioids suggests there are multiple mechanisms—then it stands to reason that whatever the theory employed, there will be some consistent effects. Even microsystems using only the ear, hand, or scalp are relied on to treat conditions as diverse as addiction, depression, high blood pressure, and stroke recovery.

Among these, auricular (ear) acupuncture[61] is the most common in the United States, perhaps because it can be easily applied to people sitting communally in chairs, either in clinical or ad hoc settings, and it has become popular among groups that treat trauma or drug addiction. Auricular acupuncture has a peculiar origin; it was developed in the 1950s, not in China but in France, by the medical doctor Paul Nogier. A branch of French medicine had developed a strong interest in acupuncture well before Mao's Communist revolution. Most notably it arrived through George Soulié de Morant, who had learned Chinese in childhood, served as a French consul in China, and received training in acupuncture in various cities where he was posted. After returning to France, Soulié de Morant was asked to translate Chinese works on acupuncture and medicine and subsequently wrote two texts of his own. A handful of physicians was also influential in bringing acupuncture to France, including Nogier, Roger de la Fuÿe, and Albert Chamfrault; the latter two gained at least some of their knowledge through military connections to Vietnam.[62]

The theory behind auricular acupuncture is based on somatotopy—specifically, on the transposition of the shape of an inverted fetus in the ear. As Hsu describes it, Nogier had a flash of insight that the antihelix of the ear corresponds inversely to the vertebral column—an insight derived from a folk healer in southeast France who cauterized a point in the ear to treat sciatic pain in her patients. According to the medical anthropologist Linda Barnes, the healer was an Algerian woman, Madame Barrin, and Nogier, intrigued, traveled to North Africa to learn more and to empirically build on his theory.[63] Hsu notes the irony of the doctor discovering [North African] folk medicine and interpreting it in terms of Western biomedicine to ultimately serve the purposes of promulgating Chinese medicine.[64] For promulgate Mao's government did: Ear acupuncture, along with scalp acupuncture and acupuncture anesthesia, were all heavily promoted during the Great Leap Forward (1958-1961) and the Cultural Revolution (1966-1976). Hsu notes that during these eras "party propaganda was at its height and learning by trial and error had precedence over deliberation and theory … acupuncture analgesia, scalp acupuncture and ear acupuncture … broke away from tradition and were allegedly discovered through practice, not theory."[65] (Perhaps coincidentally, the revolutionary detox acupuncturists would also rely on an empirical approach as they developed an acupuncture protocol to treat addiction; in their case, the dictates were practical as there were virtually no Chinese medicine texts available in English to guide them.)

During fieldwork in the late 1980s, Hsu observed that auricular acupuncture was still widely used in China because it was easy to learn, understand, and apply, and it was economical. She found that it was popular among "itinerant doctors" outside of government programs.[66] Those very reasons seem to have attracted the revolutionary acupuncturists in New York. There is no evidence they were impressed by ear acupuncture while visiting China. Rather, they came to it through an article by a Hong Kong neurosurgeon, who, while using acupuncture anesthesia, inadvertently cured his patient's opium cravings. In another example of the worlding of Chinese medicine, the technique of using ear acupuncture to treat opioid addiction made its way across cultures, a colonialist past, and a Communist revolution to land among radical activists in the South Bronx of New York.

# CHAPTER 3

# Licensed by the People: The Lincoln Acupuncture Collective

From a stage in the old auditorium of Lincoln Hospital's defunct nurses' residence, for generations one of the few places where an African American woman could earn a nursing degree, stood a jar containing up to 1,000 pills of methadone, in 40 milligram doses.[1] A mix of activists, radical young medics, and community volunteers took blood pressures, collected urine samples, and dispensed the pills to a burgeoning number of heroin users from the surrounding neighborhoods. The first people's detox program at Lincoln, created in response to the demands of the occupiers who briefly took over the hospital in November 1970, still involved methadone. However, the goal was not maintenance but tapering from maintenance. To this end, clients were dispensed progressively smaller amounts of the opioid drug.

While the program was officially part of Lincoln Hospital and thus operated under the auspices of the City of New York, it had a distinct and autonomous character. There was little communication with, or oversight from, administrators; the activists formed their own internal, collective management. Franklin Apfel recalled the atmosphere of the

*Poster advertising a benefit concert to raise funds for an ambulance for the Zimbabwe African National Union. The credit at bottom right says, "Progressive Productions of Lincoln Detox Acupuncture." Poster by Madame Binh Graphics Collective in collaboration with Mutulu Shakur.*

auditorium: "The energy and vibe were amazing. [There were] murals on the walls, music with congas and steel drums constantly ... on welfare days there was a bazaar with shops, food and clothes." Sometimes well-known performers dropped in, such as Gil Scott-Heron, the writer, poet, and spoken-word artist, who had spent his teenage years in the Bronx.[2] Scott-Heron would later participate in a benefit concert organized by the revolutionary detox acupuncture collective to buy an ambulance for the Zimbabwe African National Union (ZANU).[3] The environment described by Apfel reflects the countercultural spirit of the era, but also a sense the community was finally making Lincoln its own in some way, albeit not a seamless one.

In the beginning, methadone tapering was just one key to the detox program's approach; there was also counseling and political education. The latter part of the approach was well rooted in prevailing revolutionary therapeutic theories, which held that addiction and mental illness cannot be understood or cured by focusing on the individual alone. Some of the staff—volunteer or professional—at the detox clinic had been reading *The Radical Therapist*, a journal promoting psychological therapy as a form of liberation from sociopolitical oppression. *The Radical Therapist* decried the traditional relationship between therapist and patient as a game to maintain the power structure of society, in which women, people of color, and anyone who is different were pushed back into their subservient social roles by dominant, white, middle-class male values. Traditional therapy seen from this perspective was designed to deflect people's attention from their situation rather than to change it. Therapy "cools them out by turning their focus from society that fucks them over to their own 'hang-ups.' It puts them down by making them 'sick' people who need 'treatment' rather than oppressed people who must be liberated," read an introduction to a collection of *The Radical Therapist* articles.[4] The corrective answer was to change society: first, through educating people as to the true nature of their predicament as a product of the sociopolitical system; second, by organizing at all levels, from patient to therapist to hospital staff, to combat society's oppressive foundations. The oppressive foundations included—as had been voiced by the community mental health workers of Lincoln Hospital—professionalism. Here, *The Radical Therapist* made a clear distinction between skills and roles. It clarified the purpose of professional credentials versus practical training. One need not have professional credentials to develop successful counseling skills; professional credentials were necessary to create the role of therapist but not the skills to perform therapy, which nonprofessionals can learn.[5] The distinction remains an issue of racially inflected contention today: for example, James Doucet-Battle raises it in reference to education and treatment around Type 2 diabetes in African Americans, using the terms "expert" and "expertise" to denote siloed professionalism versus community health-worker accessibility.[6]

*The Opium Trail* likewise offered a critique of contemporary therapeutic approaches. It discussed "therapeutic communities," the most popular method of drug detoxification after methadone maintenance. Held in residential settings, the communities addressed addiction as an individual matter, although unlike methadone maintenance they focused on the psyche rather than physical symptoms. They were severely criticized for creating a rigid social atmosphere—enforcing traditional roles between the sexes, for instance—and using a strict system of reward for conformity and punishment for deviation. *The Opium Trail* concluded that the best form of therapy is a politically oriented program that first shows people how their circumstances are rooted in society, and then gives them hope and motivation to change that society. Such programs "don't deny that the individual junkie needs to change. But they understand that the best context for these personal changes, as well as the best hope for a long-range solution to the whole problem, is a mass movement fighting against racism and poverty."[7]

At Lincoln, political education had two aspects. The first was reading and discussion of revolutionary literature, of showing clients a way to view their lives as part of a broader context, one in which "they were not the problem, they were just the surplus of the economic system."[8] The second, "group therapy," organized vans to take people to courthouses to witness the trials of political prisoners.[9] While there were nationally famous political prisoners, such as Angela Davis and the BPP members known as the Panther 21, others were known only within their community of activists or protestors. A political prisoner might also be any person of color whose race or ethnicity made them likely to be arrested and charged. Political prisoners were seen as individuals who had taken on the responsibility to defend the people's human rights at the cost of their own freedom; supporting them was thus crucial to the people's fight for their dignity and equality. Many political prisoners, including Davis and the Panther 21, were eventually released, the charges against them found unsubstantiated and dropped. Over time, an increasing number of former political prisoners were recruited to the detox program as counselors. Thus, the program had a self-perpetuating political core.

As word of the community-run treatment facility spread, it became increasingly busy and soon was seeing around 25,000 clients per year. The volunteers who had been helping to run things from the outset became ever more important, trained to do intakes and collect vital signs and to help dispense methadone and other medication as well as offer social services.[10] However, business had started slowly, with only word of mouth and door-to-door recruitment to attract clients from the street. Carlos Alvarez, one of the volunteers who arrived in the first week of operations, recalled, "We took to the streets and recruited new patients by making up signs out of bedsheets that said, 'Lincoln's open.' We would go into abandoned buildings and shooting galleries, and we would just go from block to block to block to block."[11]

## Michael Smith and Mutulu Shakur

Accompanying the volunteers was a young white man, always dressed in a rumpled T-shirt, khaki trousers, and sneakers. He was often accompanied by members of the Spirit of Logos, an innovative residential anti-addiction program that had been given the stamp of approval by *The Opium Trail*, which said, "they are now doing some of the most exciting and effective anti-smack work in the country."[12] The group also published a newspaper, *White Lightning*. Some of the volunteers—most of whom were Black or Puerto Rican—took this man to be one of their own, a member of the community who liked to play 500 rum for pennies and enjoyed a game of ping pong. They were surprised to find he was, in fact, a second-year resident in psychiatry at Lincoln.[13] The man's name was Michael Smith. He was a native of southern California who had graduated from the University of California Medical School in San Francisco and become involved with the BPP in San Francisco while they were setting up free community-run health clinics. Smith had some history in New York as well; during summers while an undergraduate at Wesleyan University he had worked as a volunteer in a tutorial program in Harlem and remained in touch with the people he met there over the years.[14] While he maintained a down-to-earth persona, he had a fiery side: Smith was the doctor who had helped activists protest the death of Carmen Rodriguez at Lincoln by marching the findings of her medical chart into the hospital administrator's office. He would not shy from confrontation over the years, whether it meant responding to critics on a radio talk show attacking him for his position against the draft, or overturning tables during meetings with hospital administration.[15] To some, Smith was intimidating; others saw him as a fierce protector.[16] His former wife Debbie Smith once asked him why he wanted to be a doctor. His response was, "It isn't really that I want to be a doctor, it's that being a doctor will help me do what it is that I want to do."[17]

Smith became one of the doctors intimately involved in the detox program. From the volunteers, a few key figures would also emerge. In 1971, a seasoned activist named Mutulu Shakur joined the program. Although only 21, Shakur was steeped in revolutionary politics; he had joined the Republic of New Afrika (RNA) at the age of 17, having given the BPP serious consideration but finding the RNA more compelling. The RNA advocated for the establishment of an independent Black republic in five southern states: Alabama, Georgia, Louisiana, Mississippi, and South Carolina. At around the same age, he joined the Senate campaign committee of Herman Ferguson, an assistant school principal and the Freedom and Peace party candidate, who was running on a platform based on secession of a part of Brooklyn from the State of New York. Shakur, who was raised in South Jamaica, Queens, traveled across New York State with Ferguson, a "very, very exciting time" for the teenager.[18] While the platform—secession—was revolutionary, the campaign's modus was classic American electoral politics. The focus was a dispute over education, centering around community control of schools in the predominantly African American Ocean Hill-Brownsville section of Brooklyn.[19] Campaigning for Ferguson, Shakur was enthusiastic about the political process, and he did not see the campaign as a simple matter of Black interests against white. During the campaign, he said, "We were able to see … white people supported our right to separate and Black people supported our need to separate from the state of New York."[20]

However, the experience also cemented in his mind the limits for Black Americans in exercising their rights through the political process. Ferguson's Senate bid failed in 1968—he was convicted in the same year of conspiracy to murder two moderate civil rights leaders, including the director of the NAACP and the head of the Urban League—but the issue of secession for Ocean Hill-Brownsville continued. In March 1969, a delegation of community representatives met to discuss the matter in New Bethel Baptist Church in Detroit, where C. L. Franklin, the civil rights activist and father of singer Aretha Franklin, was pastor. Two white policemen were sent to investigate the gathering; one was shot to death, and the church was soon surrounded by police. There were reports of multiple rounds of gunshots into the church, and everyone inside was arrested. (Nearly all were later released on the orders of Judge George Crockett, Jr., an African American—an order which was bitterly contested but ultimately upheld.) Shakur, who was on security duty, recalled the church being "shot up" with "men, women, and children of all ages" inside. He later said,

At this conference and in that church at the age of 18, I became very clear that the question of separating from America, separating the Black people from America … was one of the most dangerous things that you could do … The defense of that church, the defense of those people, by members of the RNA, the Black Legion, was some of the most extraordinary—I mean heroic—show of love for a people that I had ever seen at that time.[21]

Intrinsic to the need for defense was support for political prisoners who had put their lives on the line in defense of their people. However, Shakur did not see the matter as purely one of heroic individuals or even, necessarily, of race. He spoke of the idea of a "collective protective consciousness" that encompassed not only the RNA but other Black political movements and, more broadly, the interests of all suffering peoples. With this consciousness in conjunction with individual responsibility, he said, "We will be able to bring our expectations as a people—and I'm not just talking about Black people, I'm talking about all people suffering—to bring our expectations as people to a certain level."[22] What was that level? It may have begun with the simple recognition of human dignity. Some of Shakur's earliest memories that he related to friends were of negotiating social services while being raised by a single mother who was also blind. Jackie Haught, a student and later colleague in the acupuncture colleges established by Shakur and his associates, recounted a story he had told her.

> They [social services] used to give out these commodities like Velveeta cheese, and he said they would do it right in the middle of the project, so everyone knew the poorest people in the project. And he knew it was degrading. And that they were totally about that. They weren't ever about helping anybody. He was trying to tell me that that was one of the first times he really understood what was going on.[23]

Yet Shakur's outlook was full of hope and enthusiasm. Born Jeral Wayne Williams, he claimed he had no relationship with his biological father, but as a preadolescent he found mentorship from politically active men in the community, including Herman Ferguson. These men gave him guidance and a sense of direction in life; he frequently said of himself that he was always part of a movement, and indeed the statement was almost literally true. He considered himself a dreamer, one of "the people who put into reality what we wish could happen, because they fight for it."[24] He impressed Apfel—who after leaving Lincoln became a prominent international public health advocate—as "very dynamic, very together—focused, energetic, clear thinking, an inspirational brother." Apfel added, "He was a great linker of people and I think he had quite a good analysis of what was going on around him. He was a very good organizer and worked hard to help program users understand the roots of their addictions and make lasting life changes."[25]

## Origin Stories

While the clinic was bustling with a sense of community empowerment driven by counseling and political education, it still centered around methadone. Tapering may have been an innovative use of the drug, but it was nonetheless drug use—and, according to some reports, children were sometimes accidentally overdosed. Walter Bosque recalled that by this time the form of methadone used was a clear liquid, which would be mixed with Tang, an orange-flavored drink popular in the 1970s. For days when the clinic was not open, clients would be given the mixture to take home. It would then go into the refrigerator where it could look like an appealing drink to children.[26] Coupled with awareness of this danger was the increasing sense that resolving drug addiction with drug addiction was neither effective nor desirable; in fact, it was seen increasingly as untenable. Apfel, who had been appointed medical director of the detox program in 1972—as he recalled, activist leaders went to the Lincoln doctors' collective and firmly instructed them to assign an MD to work with them—said, "There was sort of increasing concern about the use of methadone, and the amount of methadone in the community, especially related to the difficulties of methadone overdose as opposed to other opiate overdoses, because it's such a long-acting reality and because of multiple-drug abuse problems when people were using stimulants on top of the methadone."[27]

The time was ripe for an alternative—one that fit the model of community control and bypassed the paternalistic hierarchy of professionalism. It was 1972, and relations with China had been opened following President Nixon's February visit to Beijing, Hangzhou, and Shanghai. Wide-eyed stories about the success of the exotic barefoot doctors proliferated across North American newspapers. The Young Lords and other activists had been reading British physician J. S. Horne's account of being a doctor in China, including the use of acupuncture. Even in Columbia's medical school, students were exploring different kinds of Eastern body work such as shiatsu and massage.[28] Yet no one involved in the process could agree just how or when acupuncture therapy emerged as an alternative to methadone treatment for detoxification at Lincoln. Indeed, the key people in its genesis had markedly different recollections of where the idea came from and how they learned acupuncture.

Shakur and Bosque were by their account the originators of the acupuncture detoxification program at Lincoln—the Lincoln Detox Acupuncture collective, commonly known as Lincoln Detox. But even they had different memories of where they became inspired by acupuncture. Shakur recounted a personal experience from 1970, when two of his sons were involved in a car accident, leaving them with serious injuries. As Shakur described it, Yuri Kochiyama, whom he knew through political connections, took him to Chinatown. Kochiyama was involved in Asian Americans for Action, a political organization of the 1960s that was against the Vietnam war and fought against discrimination and injustice in Asian communities.[29] She was also famously photographed kneeling on the floor and supporting her friend Malcolm X's head in her hands after he was assassinated in 1965. Chinatown, Shakur said, was where "I would witness and experience the healing power of acupuncture and moxibustion for the first time in the successful treatment of my sons' traumatic brain injuries, resulting in total recovery from their paralysis and loss of speech. To me this was a miracle."[30]

Shakur affirmed that it was he who brought acupuncture to the collective. "I played a major role and I believe I did introduce the theory and principles of acupuncture, as I understood them at that time, to our program," he said. However, he emphasized that every decision was made collectively. "The collective made a decision to implement acupuncture as a modality of our overall detoxification and rehabilitation program. Each aspect of Lincoln Detox's function was governed by the collective decision-making process, involving every employee of every aspect of our program." Regarding how acupuncture was learned in its nascent days at Lincoln Detox, Shakur described what was literally a hit-and-miss process.

> We started treating people with acupuncture before we had licensing; it started by picking up books, finding points in the ear and trying it out on patients willing to give it a go in order to rid themselves of the poisons infecting their body. So we were actually doing acupuncture treatment on patients prior to developing a research protocol and prior to being licensed by the state. We were licensed by the people as this stage of therapy became, through the words and testimony of our patients, 'notorious.'[31]

Bosque, on the other hand, recalled reading an article that inspired him and Shakur to action. By 1972, Bosque said, "Mutulu and I decided that we couldn't continue to give methadone to our clients." At about that time, they came across a case study written by an acupuncturist in Bangkok, Thailand. The case reported that a man who was being treated by the acupuncturist for a non-drug-related condition confessed after his treatment was finished that, although he had been addicted to opium from the age of 12, he no longer had any desire for opium after finishing the acupuncture therapy. According to Bosque, he and Shakur immediately decided to hire two acupuncturists, who taught them the technique of auricular acupuncture, and henceforth they were able to give treatments by themselves and to train others.[32] Bosque later voiced a different recollection, of several members of the collective reading an article in the *New York Times* about Hong Kong researchers using acupuncture to treat withdrawal symptoms in heroin users.[33]

Other members of the Lincoln acupuncture collective do not remember having anyone with acupuncture expertise on the grounds in the beginning. Apfel said the doctors and volunteers learned through simply applying what they read. Generally, this meant scientific reports, as there were virtually no acupuncture textbooks or instructional guides in circulation in the United States. Apfel emphasized that the collective was always working towards finding more natural, nonchemical alternatives to methadone detoxification. "So when we saw a possible alternative option to methadone we jumped on it," he said. "We basically followed what the articles reported and adapted it to our situation. Initially neither I nor anyone in the program had any formal training." Echoing Shakur's words, he added, "We didn't have any training, or anybody come to teach us. We just read about it and then we tried to do what they said in the book and the articles, especially related to ear acupuncture. Our approach was really quite empirical."[34]

Apfel did complete a correspondence course in "Oriental" medicine, the closest thing available to acupuncture training, in which he learned some Chinese medicine theory.[35] To add "a sense of authenticity," the collective would ask a Chinese anesthesiologist who worked in the hospital—but had no knowledge of acupuncture—to sit in the room while treatments were being given. The irony of using the anesthesiologist's ethnicity to reinforce a stereotype as part of a campaign against, among other things, racism, did not register with the activists at the time. (Their rationale may have been sound, if Orientalist; the founder of the first legal acupuncture clinic in Los Angeles, Morton Barke, also observed that an "Asian aura" helped drive business.)[36] Indeed, at Lincoln, the ploy seemed to help get people to try the "new" foreign treatment. Most helpful of all in convincing people, though, said Apfel, was the effectiveness of the acupuncture itself, even in what he described as "primitivo" delivery. "We saw people come in with active withdrawal, we'd stick some needles in their ears and they would go out and play basketball. It was amazing. So once a couple of stories like that got out, it was in demand. And soon there was a core of patients promoting acupuncture."[37]

Along with James Reston's *New York Times* article, some scientific literature was trickling through to the mainstream press, including a paper by Dr. H. L. Wen and S. Y. C. Cheung of Hong Kong, published in 1973. Wen, a neurosurgeon, described a case report involving the successful, if unintended, treatment of withdrawal symptoms in a man addicted to opium. (The physicians were actually using acupuncture anesthesia to reduce pain for a scheduled surgery—the technique promulgated by Mao as a superior technique of Chinese revolutionary medicine.) Wen and Cheung then described 40 more cases of successful treatment of opioid addiction. It was the findings of this paper that were reported in the *New York Times* article cited by Bosque. The case reports, including the use of ear acupuncture and electrical stimulation, would prove influential at Lincoln.[38]

While Apfel does not remember Wen and Cheung's paper in particular, he said that after reading reports of scientific studies, "That's when we started getting into, looking at more articles and the recommendation about the electric stimulation, and we fashioned up some stimulators to plug onto the needles because it allowed us to treat more people at the same time."[39] Thus did the scientization of acupuncture, as promoted by Mao for the previous two decades and enthusiastically received by the United States in the 1970s, make its mark on Lincoln Detox.

## Danger Ahead

Despite its effectiveness, delivering acupuncture at Lincoln Detox was not for the faint of heart. This was in part because acupuncture was not all that was offered; for example, there was also the People's Program Court Collective, which provided legal aid to imprisoned poor people. The collective also helped to "organize rent strikes, building takeovers, women's health work and organization of construction workers," according to a pamphlet published by White Lightning, the self-described group of revolutionary ex-addicts who represented the white lower classes. "The people at Lincoln Detox see that all these struggles and many more are necessary before the roots of drug addiction can be ripped out of our land," the group declared.[40] Such rhetoric, coupled with the radical nature of the therapeutic approach, including counseling and political education, drew ire from certain parties on both ends of the political spectrum—and, ominously, it was not always clear from whom. As the environment became increasingly fraught, Apfel sensed danger. "There were a lot of attacks on the program from both the left and the right. There were some left-wing groups that thought it was the wrong approach to revolution and then there was the police who saw the program as a haven for terrorists. And there were a lot of infiltrators and provocateurs. So it was hard to sort things out."[41]

Eager to be reunited with his young son who had moved to the West Coast with his former wife, coupled with concerns about safety, Apfel decided it was time to leave. Although throughout his student days and medical career he had been an unrelenting activist—organizing and participating in student protests, strikes, and antiwar rallies while bucking the authority of administrators and the clout of the AMA—he no longer felt safe at Lincoln. The insidiousness of the threats created an uncertainty where people in the clinic did not know whom to trust. Apfel helped recruit Richard Taft, another young, radical doctor he knew through his Columbia contacts, to work in the program. According to Apfel, Taft had "had a problem with drug abuse in the past, and he was keen to use his past experiences in overcoming his problems to help others in a positive way." He added, "Sadly, however, months after I left, I learned that things didn't go well for him."[42]

On October 29, 1974, Taft, who had taken over as medical director of the program from Apfel, was found dead in a storage closet in the back of the auditorium in the detox building. A hypodermic syringe was next to him, but preliminary tests found no needle marks or other evidence of drug use on the "long-haired, mod-dressed doctor."[43] The time of death was estimated between 2:00 and 3:00 a.m., not a time anyone

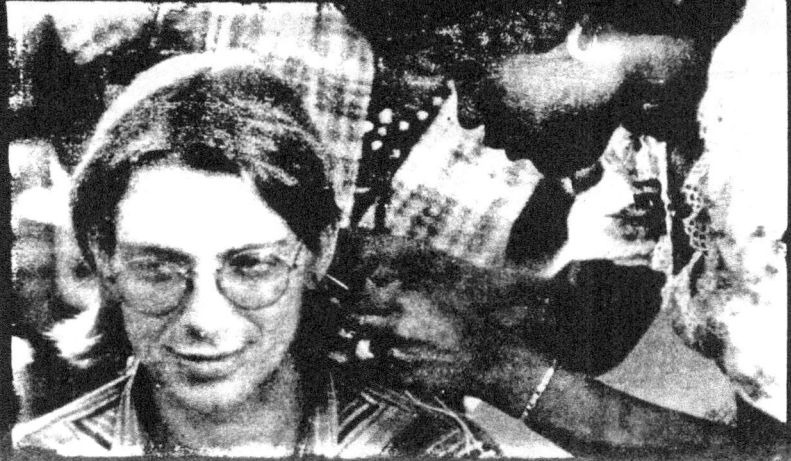

*Cover of a pamphlet published by White Lightning, the revolutionary anti-addiction organization associated with poor and working-class white New Yorkers. The photo caption says, "Richard Taft is shown here teaching another Detox worker how to use acupuncture. This is in the revolutionary tradition of a doctor using a new technique on himself before anyone else." Courtesy of the Freedom Archives.*

would normally have been in the clinic. While no one seemed to know why Taft would have been in the auditorium at that time, there were immediate suspicions among his colleagues that he had been murdered for political reasons. White Lightning and the Executive Intelligence Review (EIR) News Service both leapt into the debate from opposing perspectives. EIR was founded and headed by Lyndon LaRouche, described by the *New York Times* as "the quixotic, apocalyptic leader of a cultlike political organization." LaRouche's political leanings veered from left to right and were never conventional; an EIR edition from 2019 featured a special report headed "$CO_2$ Reduction is a Mass-Murder Policy: Designed by Wall Street and the City of London." LaRouche's political group—he ran eight times on the presidential ticket—evolved from Students for a Democratic Society (SDS), a sort of precursor to the SHO, the medical movement from which many of the radical doctors at Lincoln came. However, LaRouche's group headed in a different direction to become the National Caucus of Labor Committees (NCLC), "an organization largely made up of young upper-middle-class people who espoused Mr. LaRouche's Marxist views."[44]

The NCLC had a contentious relationship with Lincoln Detox. On May 15, about five months before Taft's death, an altercation involving the doctor and NCLC members erupted outside the clinic. According to the EIR, NCLC was holding a "press conference" outside the clinic, which it called "a brainwashing center"; White Lightning described the event as an attack against the clinic. The US Labor Party, the political party formed by the NCLC, accused Taft of "fingering" one of their members, who they described as a former intern at Lincoln Hospital, for assassination. White Lightning countered that Taft was trying to stop a confrontation at the clinic, and, moreover, that following the NCLC's accusations, Taft received threatening phone calls at his home. The argument took to television; the New York station WNEW, on its 10 o'clock news, ran a piece on the evening of Taft's death in which a clinic security officer voiced suspicion of a link between the death and the US Labor Party, according to the EIR. At around the same time, White Lightning reported, "Almost immediately after his death, NCLC said on television that Richard was a 'brainwashed zombie,' a 'CIA agent,' and 'a violent man … and it is not surprising that he met a violent death.'"[45]

However, there were other suspicions as well. White Lightning reported additional reasons Taft could have been targeted. He had given testimony on behalf of a Lincoln Hospital worker who was implicated in the killing of a transit policeman by another policeman; after the testimony, police in the courtroom made threatening gestures towards him, according to the account. It also stated that Taft had been shot at by unknown assailants, had taken to carrying a gun, and that a week before his death he had told a clinic worker that he feared for his life and wanted to take a leave of absence. The account added a final bemusing pair of details: On the day he died, Taft had been scheduled to meet "a high-ranking Washington official" to discuss funding for Lincoln Detox, but as soon as the official entered the clinic, the hospital received a bomb threat. Mutulu Shakur later held that Taft was a victim of COINTELPRO, the secret FBI counterintelligence program that targeted civil rights leaders and the Black liberation movement, among others.[46] COINTELPRO had used insidious tactics, officially since 1967 but dating back to the 1950s, to infiltrate and discredit "militant Black nationalists"—although Martin Luther King, Jr.'s nonviolent Southern Christian Leadership Conference, and King himself, were among COINTELPRO's targets. Sowing false letters of dissent and concocted evidence of immorality among group leaders, and planting agent provocateurs and infiltrators within the targeted movements, the FBI program created havoc and is credited with effectively dismembering the BPP—at which it had aimed 233 separate operations—by 1974. A lawyer who was involved in exposing COINTELPRO's operations said, "The primary focus was always the Black movement. The main problem was not that they monitored people but killed them, and set up other people to kill them." Among COINTELPRO's operations was the assassination of 21-year-old Fred Hampton, a rising star in the Illinois chapter of the BPP, in his bed in December 1969. Another young leader, Mark Clark, was also killed in the raid. It is widely believed Hampton was targeted based on the directive, contained in an FBI memo dated March 4, 1968, to "prevent the rise of a Black messiah who could unify, and electrify, the militant Black nationalist movement."[47]

For reasons that remain unclear, there was no formal autopsy report of Taft's death. The immediate cause listed on his death certificate read "pending further study."[48] Yet regardless of whether COINTELPRO played any role in the death, it contributed mightily to a rending of the fabric of political activism. As Apfel said, it was hard to know whom you could trust. Into this environment, almost immediately after Taft's death, entered Michael Smith, by now a fully credentialed psychiatrist. Legally, acupuncture could not be performed without a medical doctor in charge; Taft had been responsible for clinical oversight of the acupuncture as well as licensing and accreditation by various authorities, including the National Drug Abuse Council, the New York Addiction Service Agency, and the Health and Hospital Corporation. Smith had been working in another part of the detox program, avoiding needles. "I thought those needles were small and thin, they weren't something I wanted to do, I became a psychiatrist in order to not do these things," he said. "So I did the physicals, and I did all the other things in the program, and then one day somebody killed the doctor who was up there doing the treatment ... so it was my job to pretend that I knew how to do it, if not the program would close in 10 minutes."[49]

Smith recalled that one of the counselors—a colorful character— taught him how to do a simple acupuncture treatment. The counselor, he said, "was the model for the movie *Super Fly*, it was his biography that was made into the movie, he got royalties from it. He was a cocaine dealer, had a microphone on his car ... and pinstripes and lines of teen-agers outside his office." Smith's recollection highlights another controversial aspect of Lincoln Detox: a majority of the staff were or had been addicted to drugs—about 60 percent at the time the clinic started, by Smith's estimate.[50]

## Two Branches of Detox

Smith's entry as leader began a new era in the program—one that would lead to national recognition for acupuncture as drug addiction therapy, now known as acupuncture detox, or acudetox. It also resulted in a split between the acupuncturists who were political revolutionaries and those who were not. Mutulu Shakur was assistant director of the acupuncture program. For a while, as Lincoln Detox developed and grew, he and Smith cooperated. They even coauthored a paper on their experience using acupuncture at Lincoln. However, by the time of publication the two had long since parted ways spiritually. In recounting the successes of Lincoln Detox, they tell two separate stories while recognizing each other to a greater or lesser degree; while Shakur credits Smith with playing a critical role at one time, including putting his life and career on the line, Smith has downplayed the role of "the movement people."[51] Physically, there was a degree of separation as well. Smith, who had a dedicated team including many Puerto Ricans and African Americans, worked out of the main hospital complex. Shakur's people began formally learning and teaching acupuncture with the help of a French Canadian, Mario Wexu, from an older building several blocks from Lincoln.

While Shakur's group was also populated by Black, Latinx, and Asian Americans, there were a number of white people as well. Most of the staff, regardless of color, were invested in political activism as well as acupuncture. According to Shakur, the core of the group over the years from 1974 to 1978 included cofounder Walter Bosque from the Young Lords; Richard Delaney, an African American man who was older and more measured than most; Jennifer Dohrn, the sister of Bernardine Dohrn, who was a leader of the Weather Underground; Maria Mendoza, who had been one of the first volunteers at Lincoln Detox; Ricky Murphy—known as "the sports guy" and heavily attired in bling; and Roxanne Squire, who would coauthor a later paper with Smith. Barbara Zeller and Alan Berkman, medical doctors who were married to one another, were also core figures.[52]

Zeller, who is white, had gotten her medical degree at Columbia and knew Apfel well, along with other physicians who had joined the Lincoln doctor's collective. She joined Lincoln Detox in 1977, having already had some experience with acupuncture. In the early 70s Zeller had a friend who was having trouble conceiving; Zeller went with her to Chinatown for "behind the curtain" acupuncture treatments, the only kind available in New York. The friend became pregnant, and Zeller was so impressed that she signed up for a 50-hour acupuncture course that allowed her, as an MD, to become licensed. She was also active in support of the Black liberation and Puerto Rican independence movements, through which she had met Shakur. After having a baby of her own and leaving her job, she decided to volunteer at the clinic. Shakur told her that she could help but could not become part of the collective due to the historic distrust between white doctors and Black Americans. Nonetheless the arrangement was mutually friendly and beneficial; Zeller offered legal cover—as no one else in the clinic was licensed to perform acupuncture—and valuable advice about referring patients out for serious conditions, while she undertook in-depth study of acupuncture with a small number of others.[53]

One of these was Tatsuo Hirano. Hirano had been active in the struggle for freedom and self-determination for Asian Americans on the West coast, where he was administrator of a residential program, Asian Joint Communications, that helped Asians to get out of prison and off the streets. Like Shakur's group, the program employed political education, linking the traumas suffered by oppressed people to their entanglement in crime. It was struggling to produce results, however. Hirano met Shakur in Los Angeles in 1973 through their mutual friend Yuri Kochiyama, who had introduced Shakur to acupuncture. After hearing Shakur talk about acupuncture and its potential to "not only help detoxify and to build the health of those addicted to drugs, but to serve as a means to freedom—as a means for oppressed nationalities to free the chains of oppression," he moved to New York. By 1974 he was part of Lincoln Detox, where he began learning acupuncture skills. He related the collective's work to that of the barefoot doctors, and he saw it primarily as a sociopolitical means to free oppressed people.[54]

Another recruit was Misha Cohen, who joined the clinic in 1976. Cohen, who had been recruited by Bosque, despite being white—he told her the group was mainly Black and Puerto Rican, but they were looking for a few white people—had no experience with acupuncture, but she had been delving into alternative healing methods for some health problems of her own. She was also sympathetic to the political aspect of the program; she and Bosque had met a year earlier in Cuba, while building homes with the Venceremos Brigade, a group formed by SDS around 1970 to support Fidel Castro's socialist revolution with practical aid by Americans. Bernardine Dohrn had been closely involved with the planning of the first mission, creating another link with the acupuncture collective. When Cohen first arrived in the South Bronx clinic, she walked right into a class. "Mutulu was standing in front, and I knew I was in the right place," she said.[55] She had been studying Chinese political theory and Mao's teachings, and Shakur's explanation of the concepts of yin and yang—the opposing, interrelated forces within everything—resonated with what she knew of dialectical materialism. More than the theories, she was awed by the effects of a simple acupuncture treatment. "The very first time I saw an acupuncture treatment, I walked into a room of what looked like a hundred people who were all just totally wired. Then I watched five acupuncturists running around sticking needles in people's ears and everyone calmed down. If I hadn't already been impressed, that was it," she said.[56]

Hirano, who joined the collective two years before Cohen, described an even more dramatic scene. "People would come in with weapons," he recalled. "Because it's wild on the street. The South Bronx is like a little war zone. So people come in with their makeshift guns, knives, sticks, and you've got to leave it on the side, and you can pick it up when you leave."[57] The change in behavior after needles were inserted into the clients' ears was striking. "People come in agitated, sweating, nervous—but wanting to try. And within 10 minutes or so the room became quiet. You see people sitting there with their eyes closed. It was a very profound experience to do, to witness, and to feel the effects of it all."[58]

Lincoln Detox has become famous for having pioneered a protocol using acupuncture points only in the ear to ease addiction. Initially, treatments were given communally, with as many as 30 people seated in a circle in chairs with armrests. However, by the later 1970s Shakur's branch of the clinic used both ear and full body acupuncture to treat a panoply of ailments. There were communal rooms with chairs in which people received ear treatments, but there were also separate treatment rooms where patients lay on tables and the acupuncturists needled points on the body. The facility functioned as a community general health clinic and was constantly busy, treating anything from skin disorders to gunshot wounds. There were also occasional cases of hepatitis B. While acquired immunodeficiency syndrome (AIDS) had not yet appeared, it is probably not a coincidence that two of the acupuncture students—Cohen and Jackie Haught—would both devote a considerable part of their later careers to working with human immunodeficiency virus (HIV)/AIDS patients. The experience was "part of what so highly influenced me in terms of HIV," said Cohen. "My being at Lincoln completely guided me [in that respect]."[59]

In today's world, where acupuncture is part of many health insurance plans and can even be found in franchises, the depiction of it as revolutionary in any sense may seem hyperbolic. However, in the mid-1970s, there was more than one way in which it fit the description. First, it was a completely different approach to healthcare than the prevailing biomedical model. The traditional theory of acupuncture says that it reharmonizes systems of the body and emotions—which are inextricably interrelated—when they become unbalanced through disease or injury. Disease most often arises through extremes, of environment, diet, lifestyle, or emotion. The approach is primarily one of cultivating wellness rather than fighting illness. Shakur explained the revolutionary part in the context of drug addiction: "Remember that most drug addicts cannot conceive of anything that will make them feel relaxed and 'good' without making them feel 'high' or sedated. Acupuncture is a truly revolutionary treatment in the drug abuse field, because its effects contradict the almost universal link between being relaxed and being high. Acupuncture brings more awareness and more relaxation."[60]

But Shakur also claimed the politically revolutionary aspect. Throughout his life he has maintained that the system had a strong interest in shutting down acupuncture detox. "Our use of acupuncture at Lincoln Detox defied an entrenched history and, dare I say, confronted collusion between the pharmaceutical, political and legislative components with the military industrial complex of that era; not to mention the burgeoning prison industrial complex as aided by the ensuing war on drugs—that is the politics of it," he said.[61]

Revolutionary detox acupuncture thus embodied a paradox: on the one hand, it was a peaceful, nonviolent way of restoring a measure of sanity to people whose lives were full of conflict and violence; on the other hand, it provoked retaliation—with risk of more conflict and violence—from a deep-rooted system of power. Zeller described the clinic's political nature. "It was basically a Black and Latino collective. They were nationalist in orientation, and they were really about having the community understand the impact and the political nature of the substance abuse, of the flooding of the community with drugs," she said.[62] The politics did not diminish the devotion to acupuncture; indeed, the politics revolved around healing through acupuncture.

Revolutionary detox acupuncture took the political shapes of its era, from participatory democracy to militancy, much as did movements like the Black Panthers and Young Lords. However, while all three groups devoted considerable energy to healthcare activism, the acupuncture movement was unique in that it was centered around ideas of holistic healing. At the same time, revolutionary detox acupuncture understood healing, particularly in relation to chemical warfare, to have a political nature and a political purpose.

"We understood acupuncture as a political act," said Cohen. "For one, it was not part of anything that was part of a medical scene that existed. And it was a way to help people to free themselves from addiction, and that was seen as a political act … having people be able to stand up on their own without drugs. Think about how people feel after they get an acupuncture treatment, and the freedom from awful feelings, and feeling better, and being able to think clearly—and to connect that to a political philosophy, you can imagine how [powerful] that would be."[63]

Jackie Haught, who began studying acupuncture with Shakur in 1978, recalled that the first thing students learned about was the issue of genocide, particularly as it was carried out through chemical warfare, using *The Opium Trail* as a textbook. Initially she felt frustrated, having been eager to learn about Chinese medicine right away. However, as they began to study acupuncture, "then I really understood what it was they were trying to do, to frame the way we would be learning it," she said.[64] The frame was "understanding the long history of this country as a colonial power and as an oppressed nation of Black and Puerto Rican people that were trying to free themselves. And it was about using drugs to keep people drugged, it was about understanding that they would do anything to keep their power." Haught, who is white and comes from a working-class background, was already involved in politics but felt her eyes were newly opened. "I did not grow up the most progressive person in the world. Not somebody who went around talking bad, but I'll never forget understanding how racist my family was, and I had a lot of racism. I had to work through all this," she said.[65]

Beyond the theoretical, there was considerable practical political activity. "The whole political nature was right there," said Cohen. "[There were] always meetings of groups, there was a lot of support going on."[66] If there were a single theme, though, it would be liberation. "I think that there was a lot of different kinds of ways in which each person who was there was part of their own community's way of trying to free people in the community. And acupuncture was just one piece of it," Cohen said.[67] As Hirano described it, the core of the program's identity was that it was not just about using acupuncture to get people off drugs. Among other things, it was a continuation of the work of the RNA. He explained how acupuncture was seen as a way to serve the aims of liberation.

Having a medicine that doesn't run out, that sees the body as its innate source of pharmacy and medicine, became the most attractive form of healing at that time. For ex-slaves in this country to gain strength, you need to have self-determination, you need to have self-reliance, you need to have independence … You need to have all your basic needs being met in the highest form. And the Republic of New Afrika was the vehicle for that. So using something like acupuncture where it would help autonomy, help self-reliance and self-determination, to make the people genuinely strong, not drug dependent, became that perspective for liberation. Not the [only way], but it became part of the liberation methodology—the liberation pillar.[68]

In 1977, several members of the collective managed to travel to China on a tour given by the Chinese government. Travel was not easy to arrange because of scrutiny of Black liberation activists from the US government; when the Black Panthers went to China in 1972, they had to reroute through Tokyo at the last minute after their plane was denied entry to Vancouver. It was Haught who organized the trip, which was how she and Shakur met. Haught has a degree in psychology from Pennsylvania State University and was working as a hypertension specialist for Cornell Medical College; it was through this connection that she gained access to a tour for health workers. She was also a self-described Communist, and through political associates heard there was a group of Black revolutionaries who wanted to visit China. She and Shakur met on a street corner in Harlem. Shakur told her she should know that the CIA and FBI had blocked their previous attempts to go to China. "Then he said, 'Do you have any questions?'" Haught said, "So I said to him, 'What do you do?' and he said, 'We do acupuncture and we're starting a school.' And I said, 'Really, acupuncture, I've always wanted to do that. What is it?'"[69]

The tour, in the depths of winter just before the Chinese New Year, left a vivid impression on the travelers. Shakur, Bosque, Delaney, and Murphy joined Haught, along with a number of Puerto Rican healthcare workers from the Bronx. Haught remembered the head of the tour as a very tall Black woman who worked in a hospital in New York, where she had moved from a share-cropping family in the South. "Kids came up to her, they kept wanting to touch her hair and touch her," she said. The travelers were shown tourist attractions such as the Great Wall, but they also witnessed acupuncture. In one treatment, a doctor needled deeply into the sinus cavity of a blind man to access the optic nerve "with this very heavy-duty needle, eight to 10 inches long," said Haught. "It was amazing to watch, and the guy they were doing it to said, 'I can see a little, I can see light for the first time in my life.'"[70] They were also joined by several "white men in raincoats" who seemed to thwart interviews with the Chinese. Haught believes the men were CIA agents.

## Quebec Connection

The students were eventually able to gain full acupuncture training—not a brief course in how to needle, but a full grounding in Chinese medicine theories and practice. The training came through the father-and-son duo of Oscar and Mario Wexu. The French Canadians of Romanian descent might seem an odd choice to teach a Chinese art to a group of primarily Black and Latinx political activists; however, the Wexus' own history lent a mutual compatibility. Plus, there was a practical aspect: The Wexus ran an accredited acupuncture college, l'Institut d'Acupuncture du Quebec (Quebec Institute of Acupuncture) through which they could grant doctor of acupuncture degrees to the Americans.[71]

Oscar Wexu had fled to Paris from Romania to escape the Nazis during the Second World War. France had been developing its own branch of acupuncture since George Soulié de Morant, the French consul in China, began translating Chinese medicine texts and writing original papers on acupuncture and Chinese medicine in the early part of the twentieth century. Oscar studied acupuncture in Paris and was involved with Nguyen Van Nghi, an influential French-Vietnamese acupuncturist, and Jean Schatz, another translator of Chinese texts.[72] After moving to Montreal and starting a family, the elder Wexu founded his own acupuncture college. Father and son shared a deep distrust of medical doctors, perhaps due to Oscar's experience with the Nazis. Mario has referenced Nazis when speaking publicly about acupuncture, specifically drawing attention to the history of methadone but also accusing contemporary physicians of "experimenting" on their patients as the Nazis did.[73] He empathized with the acupuncture collective's embattled stance; describing the Wexus' experience introducing acupuncture to Canada, he said, "We were fighting the doctors. We didn't have support from anybody—just me and my father fighting the doctors."[74] Mario recalled the New York collective approaching him: "I guess they knew about the revolution we were doing. I didn't think it was a revolution—we were just having a war."[75] Most of all, Mario Wexu seemed to find a shared identity with the collective as an outsider and a nonconformist. He was also something of an expert on auricular acupuncture, as he was taking a year off to live in New York and write a book on the topic in the mid-1970s.

A relationship was soon established whereby the Wexus—mainly Mario—traveled between Quebec and New York to teach the theory and practice of acupuncture. A curriculum was developed based on the Quebec school, and Zeller taught anatomy and physiology. The courses were offered through word of mouth to people who had both an interest in learning acupuncture and a sympathetic political bent. Thus, an unrecognized, yet formal, college of acupuncture was established in Shakur's branch of the Lincoln clinic through the guidance of Shakur, Bosque, and Delaney. These three, along with a handful of others, including Ricky Murphy and Roxanne Squires, had been given scholarships by the Wexus to study in Montreal. Commuting between Canada and New York, two at a time, they received doctor of acupuncture degrees from the Quebec Acupuncture Association. Now, having returned, and with the assistance of the Wexus, they were able to grant official degrees to their students—although licensing, regulated by the State of New York, was not yet available to them. The full course offered in the South Bronx took around two years, with oral and written final exams administered by the Wexus in New York. The actual course curriculum was an eclectic mix, based on such materials as were available in English; they included mimeographs of early teachings from J. R. Worsley's Five Elements school and translations that Mark Seem—a student who would go on to found his own school, Tri-State Acupuncture College—was completing of the works of Nguyen Van Nghi, with whom Oscar Wexu had worked in France.[76]

The accredited degrees gave an important psychological boost to the collective's members. Even without licensure, the degree offered a measure of validation, proof of both professional status and evidence that the recipient had an entrée into the mysterious world of Chinese medicine, with its yin and yang, its channels and meridians, and its five phases linking everything within the human to the rhythm of the natural world. Zeller, although she had both a medical degree and a New York acupuncture license, felt particularly honored by her acupuncture degree, for she was the first medical doctor the Quebec school had allowed into its program.[77] The issue of professionalism was not simple; part of the reason for forming a school in New York was to train lay people to do acupuncture, so they could take the healthcare of the community into their own hands. Yet there was undoubtedly a measure of pride in the designation "doctor of acupuncture" for all involved. Not least, there was precious little formal acupuncture education in the United States in the mid-1970s, and Asian practitioners were marginalized "behind the curtain" as Zeller had described it—or they paid a price. Indeed, in 1974 Miriam Lee was arrested in Palo Alto, California, for practicing acupuncture without a license. In subsequent years acupuncture education would flourish, but it was a novel accomplishment in the 1970s to hold an acupuncture degree in the United States, let alone the South Bronx.

## The End of Politics at Lincoln Detox

By the late 1970s Lincoln Detox was gaining a reputation, both within New York and beyond national borders. To some viewers, the focus was primarily clinical success; to others, what stood out was the unconventional way in which success was achieved. To those focused on results, the clinic was increasingly recognized for doing effective work in combating drug addiction. Smith and Shakur prepared evidence to present to the National Hearings on the Heroin Epidemic in Washington, DC, in the summer of 1976; members of the collective were invited to the World Acupuncture Congress in Montreal the following year; and Shakur and Smith's paper was published in the peer-reviewed *American Journal of Acupuncture* in 1979.[78] The latter half of the 70s saw an increasing flow of visitors—academic and clinical—to the clinic, drawn by growing evidence of its success in treating addiction.

To others, however—namely the City of New York, the parent of the hospital and all its offshoots—Lincoln Detox was in dangerous territory. Shakur articulated both aspects of the program's reputation: "We developed predictability and we became the base of acupuncturists who were revolutionaries in this country," he said.[79] The increasing attention to the program from outsiders meant more scrutiny from the City of New York, which perhaps perceived the same thing Shakur did. The program had long been on uneasy footing with hospital administration, operating quasi-autonomously with neither blessing nor strict oversight. Against the backdrop of the controversial nature of the therapy and the presence of so many radical activists, there were official rumblings about financial mismanagement and the threat of retaliation by workers if hospital officials intervened. On November 28, 1978, on the order of Mayor Edward Koch, police surrounded the clinic building; employees were ordered to leave by Joseph T. Lynaugh, the administrator of New York City's Health and Hospitals Corporation. The unit was locked, and a sign was posted informing patients that services would be provided at the building on 140th Street. Lynaugh blamed the clinic's closure on the collective and independent nature of its management. "Politically their position was that they were independent, while our position was that they worked for the city," he said.[80] Walter Bosque, who maintained a phlegmatic attitude, said succinctly, "By 1978 Mayor Koch thought we were too radical—and he was right, we were—and they disbanded us."[81] Shakur, on the other hand, still recalls in detail every aspect of the allegations of financial mismanagement and retains a counterargument to each. He is convinced the shutdown was another attack in the ongoing chemical war. "Acupuncture in the hands of the revolutionary-minded, particularly addressing addiction, was an intervention that the government was not willing to accept at the time because it attacked and exposed the complicity of the government in imposing chemical warfare on certain segments of the community," he said. "We weren't only providing medical care and exposing chemical warfare, we were challenging Western occidental medicine by Eastern medicine and natural healing."[82]

The clinic retained a lawyer from Bronx Legal Services Inc. but was unsuccessful in fighting the allegations. Most members of the collective were reassigned to far-off posts: Vicente "Panama" Alba was sent to Bellevue Hospital, Bosque and Shakur were allocated to King's County Hospital, and Young Lords leader Mickey Melendez—who was outspoken in his comments to the press immediately following the eviction—was assigned to Jamaica Hospital. Two employees who had been key supporters of the acupuncture collective—Luis Surita, the executive director of the program, and John Lichtenstein, a medical doctor—were fired.[83] The clinic's closure marked a fateful juncture, for Michael Smith's branch of acupuncture detox continued relatively unscathed. Although formally renamed the Substance Abuse Division of the Department of Psychiatry, it continued to be known as Lincoln Detox, a name that would become famous in acupuncture and detox circles. Smith would continue to lead it for decades, further developing and propagating the acudetox technique known as NADA, which would eventually have its own organization—the National Acupuncture Detoxification Association—and earn a worldwide reputation. Revolutionary acupuncture, led by Mutulu Shakur, left the hospital and found a new home in Harlem, where it continued to merge political aims with healing, shaped by a radical vision to reform society.

# CHAPTER 4

# The Brief, Bright Life
# of BAAANA

The art of healing requires a high form of spiritual
intuitiveness. The struggle to learn acupuncture
over the last three decades within the context of
our political and philosophical view was not easy.
—Mutulu Shakur

Along a row of iconic brownstones in Harlem, up a short flight
of steps ending in a front stoop, and through a glass-framed
door hung with a pretty lace curtain were two rooms where Shakur,
Bosque, and Delaney continued to lead students in the intricate theories of acupuncture and the hard-hitting doctrines of chemical warfare
and liberation. The front room was used as a classroom, and in back
was a conference area. At street level was a clinic, with a front desk and
waiting room—sometimes doubling as a classroom—to the fore and a
treatment room behind. The so-called political people had been routed
from Lincoln Detox, but they soon had another home. Shakur, Bosque,
and Delaney formed a clinic and acupuncture school and named it the
Harlem Institute of Acupuncture, under the auspices of their newly

formed Black Acupuncture Advisory Association of North America. However, everyone referred to the college and clinic alike as BAAANA, located at 245 West 139th Street, a beautifully kept four-story brownstone in Strivers Row in Harlem.[1]

The downstairs waiting room was furnished with a sofa and a couple of chairs. Students—some of whom had followed their teachers from Lincoln Detox, and others who were newly joined—sat on the floor or the furniture during classes. In the upstairs classroom was a large conference table. Delaney, a meticulously old-school teacher, sat at the far end of the table and walked them through one of the few acupuncture texts available in English, detailing the locations and functions of one acupuncture point after another. Because books were so scarce, the students faithfully copied Delaney's lectures into their notebooks by hand; other texts consisted of xeroxed copies. If anyone found a new book on acupuncture, they shared it. "You just found things, you had to find things," said Haught. "There weren't books." Referring to theories that expand on the ordinary channels and points of TCM, she added, "I remember one day finding a book that had something to do with the extra meridians and the opening points. I can remember Mutulu being so excited about it."[2]

Education was patterned on the Quebec Institute of Acupuncture, the Wexus' school in Montreal; BAAANA operated under its wing, allowing the Harlem institute to award degrees to graduates. Some clinical experience also took place in Montreal, although not all students traveled to Canada. Students were required to provide their own white coats to wear in clinic, suggesting an interesting philosophical dynamic: On the one hand, the image of the white coat was sometimes used to connote the oppressive power of patriarchal and racist medical doctors; on the other hand, it suggested legitimacy and professionalism, attributes historically denied people of color in the United States. Here again an ambivalent attitude to professionalism was evidenced; professionalism was criticized when it was used to deny lay people the right to take control of their own healthcare, but when it became accessible to lay people—as through the doctor of acupuncture degree—it was embraced as a brand of legitimacy, a symbol of equal power.

Clinic services were free or priced on a sliding scale. Through word of mouth the Harlem clinic became a busy place, and the more advanced students quickly gained experience. They performed full-body acupuncture, based partly on TCM, the standardized form of acupuncture developed under Mao's government. But there were other influences as well, namely an energetic understanding of the medicine that may have come from the Wexus—the elder Wexu had learned acupuncture in France from scholars whose work was published prior to TCM, and where Nogier's system of auricular acupuncture was developed. One of the practices that came from the Wexus was a form of massage along the acupuncture channels, given to clients by the less experienced students before the acupuncture treatment. While some students recalled being trained to competently perform basic acupuncture, others described a more sophisticated style. Karen Cutler, who had to redo much of her training after moving to California—which has its own requirements and exam for licensure—said, "The education in California was very strict TCM and my education in New York was not TCM. In New York, there was a lot of five-element theory and, in the last year, a primary focus on the energetics of meridian theory. I found it [California] so stifling. I was very aware of the value of what I'd learned at BAAANA. I'd internalized the spirit of the medicine in a way I don't think it was ever communicated or emphasized during my educational experience in the 90s at my acupuncture college in California."[3]

In contrast to Delaney's staid teaching style, Shakur could be inventive and inspirational. Especially in the absence of textbooks, he employed lived experience as a learning tool. One night, early in the second cohort's training, the students sat around the large table in the upstairs classroom. They had been learning about the concepts of yin and yang, embodying female and male, dark and light. Shakur walked in and turned off the ceiling lights, plunging the room into darkness. "We sat there in a dark room—we sat there what felt like a long time but was probably no more than five minutes," recalled Cutler. "It was very abrupt—first he blackened the room and we all just sat there quietly, a bunch of people sitting around this table for five minutes in silence. It creates a certain mood, and then BOOM! The lights came back on. It was kind of brilliant, very experiential. It was his way of teaching us yin and yang. He wanted us to talk about what it felt like—sitting in a dark room, and then that transition to the bright lights. And it was just a very enlightening exercise."[4]

In the clinic the students were seeing a range of disorders going well beyond addiction. "We had plenty excitement," recalled Haught. "We treated people crippled by gunshot wounds. I remember all these Black celebrities came." She added, "But it was never, ever done out of the context of human rights and the right of community control of medical services."[5] Haught's point speaks to the raison d'être of the clinic: It had an overt political purpose, but it was genuinely invested in obtaining its goals through providing affordable healthcare by using an Eastern form of healing that could be learned and employed by people in the community. Both politics and healing were clearly in evidence at BAAANA. "You couldn't walk into that clinic without seeing the posters on the wall. I think the primary purpose was to train people as acupuncturists, but the whole thing was a political program, in the middle of everything else that was going on in the community," said Zeller. "There were posters, they were doing work around political prisoners, it was a political place. I don't think there was an introductory thing about it, 'If you come to this school …,' but the focus was on the role acupuncture could play [in larger political spheres]."[6]

At the same time, not all the students were political; some came simply to learn acupuncture. There was as yet little formal acupuncture education in the United States, and BAAANA was less expensive than most acupuncture colleges. Karen Cutler arrived as a 26 year old with a theater arts degree and an interest in Kundalini yoga. She had become enamored of acupuncture after being treated successfully for a whiplash injury at Lincoln Detox. Cutler was aware of the revolutionary nature of BAAANA but was not drawn to the politics. "We had as a huge part of our education, and they were very upfront about it, political education," she said. "The whole idea was to expose the persecution and oppression of the people in the community through the systemic use of drugs. Mutulu was a political activist—he was a revolutionary … It was his vision to educate in Chinese medicine and revolutionary thought. And practicing acupuncture was pretty revolutionary at that time."[7]

Other students were attracted to BAAANA by both the political vision and the acupuncture. One of these was Urayoana Trinidad, who, like Haught and Zeller, had come from Lincoln Detox after the closure. Trinidad was a clinical psychologist who held a master's degree in clinical and community psychology and had been working in hospitals and community facilities in the Bronx and the East Harlem neighborhood known as El Barrio. She had long been involved in the struggles at Lincoln Hospital, including the 1970 takeovers. A Puerto Rican, she was married to an African American man. She was quietly but fiercely political, an intellectual—Shakur said of her that she had "always been cerebral, allowing her mind to dictate her destiny"—who was profoundly respected by other students.[8] Trinidad tended to dress all in white, traditional Yoruban clothing; her dark brown hair was pulled back with a decorative piece, sometimes paired with an arresting necklace. Students and faculty alike respected her distinctive style and deliberate, exacting manner. Anne Lown recalled, "She was an incredible leader. I think she was deeply political but never discussed politics when I was with her."[9] Later, when things began coming apart, Trinidad would become the solid center, holding the vision of acupuncture education together.

There were also white students who were dedicated revolutionaries. Most were members of the May 19th Communist Organization or its offshoot, the Madame Binh Graphics Collective (MBGC). May 19th—so named for the birthdates of Ho Chi Minh and Malcolm X and the anniversary of the death of José Marti, a leader in Cuba's fight against Spanish rule—had evolved from the Weather Underground Organization, which itself had evolved from SDS. Self-described as a small, anti-imperialist, "Marxist-Leninist 'cadre' organization that was based in New York City from 1977 to 1983," May 19th was comprised of white revolutionaries who supported Black and brown liberation movements, particularly in Africa, Cuba, and the United States.[10] The MBGC was a still-smaller collective of white women artists, many of them lesbians, who created posters, prints, and street art in tandem with the larger goals of May 19th. Both groups wrestled with a deep inner conflict rooted in their belief that being white was an irremediable source of damage to the society they envisioned—and there was only slight succor in belonging to other oppressed categories. Mary Patten, a former MBGC member, who was not involved in BAAANA, wrote,

> We had a very hard time representing white people in struggle, because our analysis dictated that whites were almost irredeemably tied to the imperialist system. We viewed every chapter in the white working class struggle in the U.S. ... as defined by white supremacy and betrayal. We saw every expression of solidarity from the white-dominated left ... as marred by racism ... a burden that could only be overcome by ascribing to and participating in our vision of "war in amerikka," the willingness to sacrifice *everything* to become revolutionary allies. ... For a period, we believed that white women, especially white working class lesbians, were the "weak link" in the white oppressor nation and thus the most likely to be allies of national liberation struggles.[11] [Emphasis in original.]

May 19th was one of a large number of small revolutionary entities, many of whom overlapped at times. Shakur, a great networker, was involved in various movements supporting political prisoners and Black liberation. There was thus inevitable communication between BAAANA and other groups, which were going through their own metamorphoses; by the late 1970s, for instance, the BPP and the Young Lords were effectively gone, partly if not entirely through the undermining work of COINTELPRO. Patten's writing suggests what the attraction to BAAANA may have been for her cohort: "In May 19th and the MBGC, we were always imagining a cascading, ever-growing force of Black people whom we saw as central to the process of revolutionary change in the US—seizing their own destinies, and, in the process, rescuing us from ours."[12] The racial makeup of the school reflected the complexity of the movement—acupuncture as revolution—and of the broader environment of liberation, in which organizations evolved and dissolved, formed alliances and split bitterly, while the Black liberation movement generated fervent white supporters. The power imbalance between white Americans and African Americans created a further conundrum: Many of the lawyers representing Black political prisoners were white; so were most of the radical doctors who supported the Young Lords and other activists during the takeovers at Lincoln. Fitzhugh Mullan wrote of the phenomenon of guilt experienced by the doctors, a feeling carefully picked apart and criticized at collective meetings.[13] The self-effacement by May 19th surpassed even the self-criticism of the doctors, however. Patten analyzed the way MBGC members tried to make their whiteness invisible by creating anonymous poster works, or by attributing the poster to the liberation group for whom it was made.

There is nothing wrong, and a lot "right" with this, in principle: it's a solidarity gesture. But what needs to be scrutinized, in our case, is the act of inflating the apparent visible support that existed for certain revolutionary tendencies of the Black Liberation movement at the time, and in the process, the attempted erasure of our whiteness. Our insistence that white people had no escape route from the trappings of white privilege, no other avenue to becoming revolutionary, than to "go to war," was an attempt to "disappear" into the imagined masses of the Black Liberation Struggle.[14]

There was thus a mix of motivations at BAAANA, held by people who were Black, white, and Puerto Rican (and, in Hirano's case, Japanese American) and who had various conceptions of revolution and varying degrees of commitment to it. The unifying force that held it all together, for a while, was the belief that acupuncture was a revolutionary, compelling, and effective way to realize the goal of community-controlled healthcare available to all. However, to many involved at BAAANA, the goal of acupuncture as a vehicle for the liberation of oppressed peoples was preeminent. The fundamental understanding of the role of drugs in the community, as financed and supported by the government, was also a linchpin principle. For his part, Shakur had always been open to working with whites as part of the Black liberation movement; as a teenager working for the RNA, he had learned to see a clear distinction between separatism and racism.[15] Among the projects on which he coordinated intimately with whites was the National Task Force for COINTELPRO Litigation and Research. Cofounded by Shakur while he was still working at Lincoln Detox, the task force was established to expose the extent of attacks by government agencies, through COINTELPRO, against progressive organizations. Included on its advisory board were the congressman Ronald Dellums, an African American, and intellectual Noam Chomsky, of Russian-Jewish descent and at the time a Massachusetts Institute of Technology professor. Among the staff attorneys was Susan Tipograph, a New York lawyer, who was white and who would later act as legal advisor to Susan Rosenberg, one of the more revolutionary students at BAAANA.[16]

After three years of operations, with the second cohort of students firmly entrenched, BAAANA was raided by the FBI. It was March 26, 1982. Cutler, who had taken the train from Brooklyn on the way to her clinic shift, rang the doorbell as usual but there was no response. "I ring the bell a second time and someone pulled the lace curtain aside and shows the badge of the FBI," she recalled. "I saw all these local tv trucks outside on the way there, and I thought 'Oh, they're doing a program on our school.' They showed the badge and said, 'School is closed today.' I turned around and all those tv cameras were on me."[17]

The FBI had unleashed a sweeping series of raids to track down anyone implicated in the armed robbery of a Brink's truck in Nanuet, New York, about 25 miles north of Manhattan, on October 20, 1981.

A Brink's guard, Peter Paige, and two policemen—Waverly Brown and Edward O'Grady—were killed in the act, deemed an "expropriation" of $1.6 million by the perpetrators, a group identified with the Black Liberation Army and Revolutionary Armed Task Force.[18] Caught up in the FBI's net were numerous people associated with BAAANA, including clinic and other staff. Many were subpoenaed and some were jailed for refusing to testify in front of a federal grand jury, including Trinidad's husband, who was to spend nearly three years in prison for his stance. Shakur went underground. The FBI alleged that BAAANA "served as 'headquarters' for the Brink's gang and a 'communications center' for a network of safe houses that stretched from coast to coast."[19] A federal grand jury was impaneled to determine whether the Brink's robbery was part of a pattern of racketeering involving other violent actions by revolutionary groups. Not least among these actions was the prison escape of Assata Shakur, a famed political prisoner whose subsequent free life in Cuba was seen as a perpetual black eye on US law enforcement. (Previously known as Joanne Chesimard, Assata Shakur adopted her name, as did Mutulu Shakur, as a personal and political statement.)[20] The FBI would eventually use the Racketeer Influenced and Corrupt Organizations (RICO) Act to charge individuals it believed were connected to the Brink's robbery, including Shakur.

BAAANA was rent apart by the FBI raid. Delaney left and eventually moved to the Southwest, where he would spend the next decades of his life quietly practicing acupuncture, until his death in 2019. One student recalled, "Everyone was mad at him for a while," after his departure. But another said, "Richard took on a teaching role, and I think he was being relied upon a lot. Because he was very dedicated, dedicated to passing the information that he had along, just dedicated as a teacher. My sense was when things were getting hot politically, he wanted to leave."[21] Haught had also left, after earning her degree, disconcerted by the direction the politics had taken. "[At] BAAANA I met a lot of real revolutionary forces who came through there all the time, and that wasn't a good thing. It should not have been like that," she said. Speaking of the acupuncturists, including Shakur, she added, "Because they weren't good at waging war, they weren't trying to be soldiers, they weren't like the CIA, they were just trying to make the world better."[22] She moved to the Pacific Northwest where she practiced acupuncture and helped a naturopathic college set up an acupuncture program. From afar, she watched the Brink's catastrophe unfold on television, people she knew handcuffed and escorted to jail. She refused to speak to the FBI agents who cornered her off and on, trawling for information. For May 19th, the Brink's robbery marked "the beginning of the end," as the recently formed FBI-New York City Police Department Joint Terrorist Task Force moved to crush radical movements of all colors.[23]

Contributing to the chaos at BAAANA were the actions of a man who had been with them from the days at Lincoln Detox. Known first as Peter Middleton, then as Kamau Bayete, he had carried a lot of administrative responsibilities but had no authoritative power. Initially Bayete defended the school after the raids, standing on the steps of the federal courthouse at Foley Square in Manhattan to tell reporters, "Our reputation has been slandered. A lot of our patients are afraid of being subpoenaed on the spot, like we were."[24] However, 14 months later he gave testimony against other defendants, stating that he had previously lied to FBI agents and admitting that he was a "heavy user of cocaine."[25] The FBI alleged that surveillance showed he had regularly bought cocaine from a dealer on the same block as BAAANA. Bayete's testimony, though, centered not around drugs but on activities of other defendants accused in the Brink's robbery. One of them, Silvia Baraldini, was a May 19th member who was not affiliated with BAAANA; the summer before Bayete's testimony—not long after he had defended the school on the courthouse steps—the MBGC distributed a poster with Bayete's likeness on it, labeled "Wanted— Dead or Alive." The FBI later depended on Bayete to interpret "cryptic" conversations it had recorded from wiretaps at BAAANA during three and a half months of surveillance.[26]

The most dedicated acupuncturists at the school were scathing in their response to Bayete and the FBI. "He did this absolutely on his own because as you know we consider the use of drugs to be chemical genocide," said Trinidad of Bayete, speaking at a press conference in September 1982.[27] Zeller accused the Joint Terrorist Task Force of acting for political reasons. "BAAANA was targeted by the Joint Terrorist Task Force because it is a revolutionary institution, capable of enabling the New Afrikan Nation to resist genocide and fight for its liberation," she said at the press conference, which was held in Harlem to protest impending hearings in the case.[28]

The abrupt, forceful closure of BAAANA following the Brink's "expropriation" marked the end for revolutionary detox acupuncture. Militant direct action had by now proved untenable against the power of the state for those leftist groups who engaged in it in the early 1970s. Indeed, most of them did not survive the decade, split apart by factionalism, financial woes, and police and FBI violence.[29] The acupuncture movement was no different in that sense. If acupuncture were to continue to pursue some form of revolutionary agenda, it would have to abandon political declarations.

## First World Acupuncture: The Movement Reborn

Even as the Joint Terrorist Task Force pursued its case, Trinidad maintained her vision for acupuncture, while raising her children alone as her husband remained in prison. In January 1983, the school and clinic reopened—or, more accurately, were reborn—with a new name and an altered focus. Trinidad also had a birthing practice, and the acupuncture school moved into the same location, a more modest brownstone than the Strivers Row building, at 354 West 123rd Street, not far from Columbia University. Officially named the Institute of Traditional Chinese Medicine of New York City, under the auspices of the First World Acupuncture Advisory Association, the enterprise was known colloquially as First World Acupuncture. The name was used to counter the bitter history of so-called Third World peoples at the hands of medical systems, as the course catalog explained:

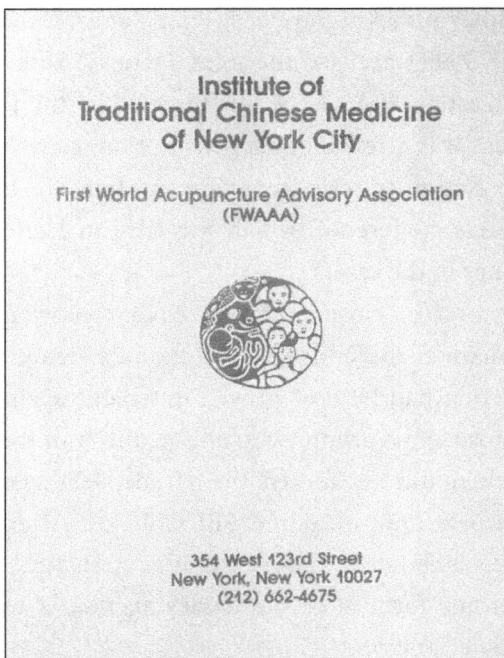

*Cover of the course catalog for the Institute of Traditional Chinese Medicine of New York City, commonly known as First World Acupuncture, circa 1983. Courtesy of Jackie Haught.*

"Third World" people in the US have been forced to accept humiliation, experimentation, sterilization, surgical and chemical abuse by the US health care system and its institutions. We use the term "First World" to honor the ancient practices and development of the cultures in the Americas, Africa, and Asia ... In modern times, these nations are most commonly referred to as "Third World" due to their deliberate underdevelopment by Europe.[30]

The clinic at First World Acupuncture functioned similarly to the one on 139th Street. Every patient was first examined by a senior acupuncturist, who went through the diagnostic ritual of pulse-taking and tongue exam before devising a plan for treatment. Next, a student would perform acupressure and other massage along the acupuncture meridians (specified regions of the body on which points are typically needled). Finally, an acupuncture treatment was given by one of the acupuncturists, all of whom had graduated from one of the two schools. As at BAAANA, the clinic was widely used by the community and was nearly always busy. Acupuncture was still a novelty in New York, but the sign out front advertising acupuncture services roused attention. It was the kind of place where a neighborhood resident struggling with mental, physical, or addiction issues might climb the stairs to find out what lay beyond the clinic doors and, if lacking the resources to pay for treatment, might work out a barter system doing secretarial work in exchange for acupuncture. There was among such patients a feeling of being cared for by a community. They found the people who spoke to them and worked with them were not like the doctors they were used to; the clinic felt like a safe place, the acupuncturists more like friends than disinterested authority figures.

Like BAAANA, the new school was accredited to offer degrees. As a member of the American Association of Acupuncture and Oriental Medicine and the Acupuncture Coalition of New York, as well as the Quebec Association of Acupuncture and the International Association of Traditional Chinese Medicine, it became one of only 11 institutions in the United States, Canada, and Europe accredited to teach traditional Chinese medicine.[31] In contrast to BAAANA, however, it was focused only on teaching acupuncture and providing treatments to the community; any overt sign of politics was gone. The mission of the institute was fundamentally one of radical change, though.

As the center of a movement, First World Acupuncture was most notable for its role in North American acupuncture education. Among its stated goals were to train acupuncturists to meet the health needs of underserved communities through establishing a self-reliant health-care system based on natural medicine alone, "to enable us to promote the health of our people," and to "promote a non-chemical permanent solution to chemical genocide (heroin, methadone, alcohol, cocaine, etc.), which is killing and paralyzing huge numbers of our people."[32] The school also declared its support for the universal human rights "of all people to choose and control their health care," and "of all oppressed people, in particular Black and Latino people, to be trained in acupuncture and other forms of traditional medicine."[33] And it took the unprecedented step of offering a Traditional Acupuncturist in Service to the Community degree.[34]

The spirit recalls that of the barefoot doctor program—as widely perceived by global public health authorities in the 1970s—in its mission to reach China's profoundly underserved rural populace. For decades, no acupuncture college in the United States offered a similar degree; indeed, education went generally in the opposite direction, becoming increasingly expensive and, partly as a result, encouraging graduates to focus on a wealthy clientele or biomedical integration. Not until 2014, with the founding of POCA Tech by the People's Organization of Community Acupuncture, has another acupuncture college focused on producing graduates dedicated to community service. In this sense, First World Acupuncture laid the foundation for revolutionary changes in acupuncture education—a struggle that continues today.

At the new college in Harlem, Barbara Zeller maintained her interest in the project as executive director of health services. Like Trinidad, she had suffered personal sacrifices for her beliefs and was now a single parent; her husband, the physician Alan Berkman, would go underground for two years, with members of the May 19th Communist Organization, after being subpoenaed to appear before a grand jury on suspicion of having given medical treatment to a suspect in the Brink's robbery. He subsequently spent eight years in prison for convictions related to the possession of matériel and literature in connection with revolutionary activism.[35] Haught returned, having left May 19th and feeling that she was making amends for her abrupt departure, and believing strongly in the renewed mission to focus on acupuncture and healthcare as a human right. "I knew I had to figure this out," she said. "I couldn't leave it be the way it was, and I still really believed in what was trying to be done."[36] Cutler and other students followed when they learned the school was opening; she and a few others eventually joined the faculty as new students arrived. Some of them came out of interest in the radical approach to healthcare; some had heard of First World through political associates. But political talk was muted.

"There was nobody there who was apolitical," said Anne Lown, who had not been at BAAANA. Lown, who became a researcher in the psychosocial consequences of trauma and an associate professor at the University of California, San Francisco, added, "But some people were more and less engaged in politics. Everybody was acting from what I think was a radical point of view—though we did not discuss politics there much at school. None of us did. There were a lot of women in our class, and we talked about our kids a lot. We talked a lot about acupuncture, and what made us and others better, and how to provide acupuncture."[37]

Karen Cutler saw a clear distinction from the days at BAAANA. "I think the focus of the politics at that point [after First World opened] was really around providing healthcare. I think the politics when we were up on 139th Street was about politics for the sake of the politics. And that's not to say they weren't dedicated to teaching us, but I think Urayoana was really much more focused on educating us about Chinese medicine. Even though her politics were clear her energies as an educator were more directed to the Chinese medicine curriculum. That is not to say we didn't learn a lot about Chinese medicine theory at BAAANA because we studied a lot—we had lectures, exams, clinics, etc.—but the undercurrent was the political education."[38]

"Urayoana was just really focused on healing, and her community, and taking good care of people in the community, and providing the best possible acupuncture and medical care," said Lown. "She did not wax eloquent about her politics ever, from what I heard … Mutulu was much more of an explicit political leader. And Urayoana was a leader by practice, by providing, by having the school, by providing the clinic for the community."[39]

The facilities were still fairly rudimentary, although the brownstone, smaller than the one on Strivers Row, was nonetheless beautiful. And it had another attraction: In the basement a volunteer ran an informal eatery, stir-frying greens and other healthful foods. On the first floor was the main room of the school. This time there were not even chairs—the institute ran on a shoestring budget, financed by a sliding-scale clinic and low-cost tuition—so the students, who were mostly in their twenties, sat cross-legged on the floor. Tuition ran to $5,175 (around $14,330 in 2021 dollars) for the three-year program, with a few work scholarships offered based on need and a commitment to work with underserved Black and Latinx communities. There were one or two textbooks, and an anatomy coloring book for learning anatomy, taught by a massage therapist. As before, there was a strong reliance on photocopies. One fall day in 1983, one of the students came in excitedly waving a book; Ted Kaptchuk's *The Web That Has No Weaver* had just been published, and some of its contents would be used in the inaugural National Commission for the Certification of Acupuncture (NCCA) exam the following spring. Kaptchuk gained enduring renown in the world of Western acupuncture on the basis of the book, a seminal work laying out the origins, philosophy, and practice of Chinese medicine.[40] The book proved crucial, as some of the information on the NCCA exam had not been taught at either BAAANA or First World Acupuncture.

It is not clear if the students were aware that Kaptchuk's own radical history led him to study acupuncture, but several would eventually complete a two-year course in Chinese herbology with him. Kaptchuk had been very active in radical left politics during the late 1960s, when he was a student at Columbia University. After graduating with a degree in East Asian Studies in 1968, he was sought by the FBI to testify before a grand jury in connection with political activities. He took refuge in a commune belonging to the San Francisco Red Guards—a group inspired by the Red Guards, paramilitary bands of students who helped Mao purge "revisionists" from the Communist party during the Cultural Revolution—in California, where he came across information on Chinese medicine. In 1970, after leaving the commune, he studied with Dr. Hong Yuan-bain, a student of Cheng Dan'an, the man credited with reviving acupuncture and giving it a scientific founding during China's Republican era.[41]

Kaptchuk's goal was to further his studies in China. However, his entrance was thwarted by Sino-American relations prior to the Nixon era. He asked friends among the Black Panthers who were traveling to China to take a letter to the Chinese government on his behalf, requesting help for access to mainland China for his study. Eight months later he received a reply, stating that people with American passports couldn't study in Chinese schools.[42] In lieu of China, he spent two years learning with Dr. Hong followed by two years studying in Taiwan. Following these, he took on a three-year course and apprenticeships at the Macau Institute of Chinese Medicine, where he earned his Chinese medicine degree. Kaptchuk returned to the United States in 1976 and joined the faculty at the newly formed New England School of Acupuncture, the first formal acupuncture school in the country. In 1990, he joined the faculty at Harvard Medical School, a rare expert in what was then called "alternative medicine" at one of the pillars of Western medicine.

In the ensuing decades, Kaptchuk has become a part of that pillar himself, as a professor of medicine and director of a prestigious research institute. While his path to acupuncture began in the same earth as that of the radicals who formed Lincoln Detox and BAAANA, there was a key difference in his role as a white, middle-class male. He too recalls discussion of the barefoot doctors and the excitement they generated among leftist political groups. His decision to study Chinese medicine stemmed partly from interest in its philosophy, but also from Mao's politics. "I could have chosen Ayurvedic medicine or Unani medicine but the fact that a left-wing government and Song dynasty philosophy both supported Chinese medicine lent more attraction to going to China," he said.[43]

There was one aspect of clinic work that was frightening to some students at First World Acupuncture. In 1982 the Centers for Disease Control and Prevention introduced the acronym AIDS to the medical lexicon; over the next few years, the disease would run rampant through populations of gay men and intravenous drug users in the United States. The single-use disposable needles that are universally employed by American acupuncturists today were not yet in use. Instead, needles were reused after being cleaned in an autoclave or pressure cooker. "We would put them into these little containers that should turn blue when the temperature gets high enough to say that this should be sterilized," explained Lown. "But God knows it was at the height of the AIDS epidemic. When we were practicing, we had to practice on each other, and the students were not comfortable. And we thought, 'What do we do? This is what we're doing for people in the community.'" When a decision was made to use a single-use style of needle, everyone was relieved.[44]

There were no needling disasters and no FBI raids. Yet First World Acupuncture survived only a handful of years. The reasons were fairly mundane in the end. As more acupuncture schools around the country opened, licensure became more closely scrutinized. While graduating students could take the NCCA exam, they still could not obtain an acupuncture license in New York without having either a medical degree or proof of 10 years of practice elsewhere. Moreover, the finances were not working out; everyone was just scraping by. "I don't think I ever made any money at First World," said Haught. "It barely paid the bills. And it consumed my life."[45] Students were having babies and raising families, moving on. The school closed its doors by 1984. Shakur remained underground until February 1986 when he was apprehended by the FBI in California. He was indicted under RICO, and in 1988 a jury comprised of seven African Americans, three Latinx people, and two white individuals found him and codefendant Marilyn Buck "guilty of conspiracy to violate the Racketeering [sic] Influenced and Corrupt Organizations Act, participation in a racketeering enterprise, bank robbery, armed bank robbery, and bank robbery murder," although no evidence at trial found that he killed anyone.[46] Shakur was sentenced to 60 years in prison.

It appeared that it was up to the graduates of First World Acupuncture and BAAANA to carry on the spirit of revolutionary acupuncture. The political revolution had collapsed in on itself under pressure from numerous sources, including fallout from the Brink's robbery, the continuing threat of the FBI, the growth of acupuncture education in the United States, and broader social changes. Over the decades to come, some alumni of the two colleges would continue to use acupuncture to "serve the people." Their focus on relief for the most marginalized in society found new outlets as HIV/AIDS spread. Other individuals who had worked with Michael Smith at Lincoln Detox also set out to use acupuncture to address drug addiction or trauma. In Oakland, California, the physician Tolbert Small, informed by his visit to China and a long commitment to the struggle for civil rights, continued to provide acupuncture to the African American community. The influence of these practitioners has made incremental inroads into the practice of acupuncture in the United States. However, it did so in a largely apolitical manner, far from talk of revolution, until the advent of POCA.

CHAPTER 5

# Acupuncture for the Masses: The People's Organization of Community Acupuncture

In February 2012, Lisa Rohleder, an acupuncturist and entrepreneur living in Portland, Oregon, stirred up the normally sedate waters of the *Journal of Chinese Medicine* (*JCM*) with an article accusing the majority of acupuncturists in the Western world of being disconnected elitists. The *JCM*, which is published in England, was founded in 1979 by Peter Deadman, a pioneer of Chinese medicine in the UK. Deadman, now a senior figure in international acupuncture circles, is still the coeditor of the *JCM*, where he normally remains behind the scenes, aside from conducting an occasional interview for the journal. He is perhaps best known in the United States as the coauthor of *A Manual of Acupuncture*; the tome, published in 1988, is widely used as a textbook and may be the closest thing there is to a bible for students at many US acupuncture colleges. In this case Deadman, having accepted the article for publication, was moved to respond, in the next issue, with a sharply worded rebuke arguing that Rohleder's vision of acupuncture risks "impoverishing Chinese medicine," and that if it were adopted as the mainstream model, the "cost—the loss—[would be] too high."[1]

Wading into journalistic confrontation was not new to Rohleder, who in 2006 was fired as a columnist at *Acupuncture Today*, a US trade publication that mainly serves as an uncritical disseminator of news and an advocate for the industry, because the editors thought her column had "dangerous potential."[2] Rohleder thrives on such challenges and on the image of dangerous potential; she has referred to her world, sardonically, as "the dark side."[3] *Acupuncture Today*'s alarm may have been based on the online response to Rohleder's columns: They tapped into an underground swell of discontent with the profession by a previously silent minority, who latched onto her ideas in vehement forum posts, eventually leading to an organization of like-minded acupuncturists calling themselves "punks."

The columns, which continued for a year, began innocuously enough with philosophical and practical discussions of social entrepreneurship—the idea that business can be a tool to solve social ills as well as being socially and environmentally responsible. In her first piece, Rohleder laid out her vision for the role of acupuncture in society:

I believe the heart of acupuncture is radical, elegant simplicity. Because of this, acupuncture is extraordinarily flexible. It can adapt to any treatment setting, any practitioner and any culture, while remaining remarkably effective. As years passed … I became possessed by a vision of what acupuncture could do for the problems of our health care system as a whole. Imagine what could happen if acupuncture were widely available to everyone in America, regardless of whether they had insurance or not. Imagine the impact of a clinic in every neighborhood: patients getting off expensive pain medication they can't afford, uninsured asthma patients no longer needing to go to the ER, overwhelmed working parents no longer yelling at their kids or drinking to escape from the stress of their lives—because they have an alternative. Imagine acupuncturists being integral to every community, and acupuncture being the medicine everyone uses and values.[4]

By her last two articles, Rohleder was overtly questioning the dominant model of acupuncture and placing her model, which she calls community acupuncture, as a paradigm for social change and social justice. Her last column was about power and privilege.[5] She homed in on the privilege of being part of the middle class, which she did not have as a child and has never been able to identify with since. Her vision of society was strongly shaped by the poverty of her upbringing, which has also defined her view of the business of acupuncture. As evidenced in the name of her flagship clinic, Working Class Acupuncture (WCA), much of her focus is on accessing—or making acupuncture accessible to—people of the working class. Her penultimate column used an extended analogy of the early automobile industry, ending with a contrast between selling Cadillacs versus Model Ts. Do acupuncturists want to woo the relatively few who can afford luxury or offer an effective workhorse that most people with a job can afford? Is their mission about attracting the most money or the most people in need?

The *JCM* article, titled "Community Acupuncture: Making Buckets from Ming Vases," changed the analogy to one both more culturally attuned and far more stinging to the world of Chinese medicine. In choosing the Ming vase as a metaphor, Rohleder craftily alluded to the tendency of Western acupuncture clinics to use Chinese art and images in their décor; while she did not use the term in the article, her image evokes Chinoiserie, originally a fanciful European interpretation of Chinese art and design popular in the seventeenth and eighteenth centuries but now also understood as a subgenre of Edward Said's Orientalism.[6] The bucket, in contrast, is an unpretty but useful object that anyone can have. In Rohleder's description, mainstream acupuncturists hold out their expensive education as they would a Ming vase, as something exotic, rare, and valuable, and expect to be rewarded for it in terms of income and social status. The bucket is what the Ming vase becomes—or was in the first place, in the way of *The Emperor's New Clothes*[7]—when community acupuncturists use it to hold vast quantities of the water they pour over people in need of quenching.

Rohleder is a prolific writer, and she has published, online or in print, several works that could be labeled manifestoes (one of the first is called *The Little Red Book of Working Class Acupuncture*). The Ming vase article has the touch of a manifesto as well, defining community acupuncture, punks, and the kind of person the movement wants and doesn't want, as well as enumerating the important aspects of her business model. Noting the varied definitions of punk as a substance that will smolder and light things, an unimportant person or ruffian, and someone characterized by defying social norms of behavior, she writes,

> Community acupuncture needs people who are able and willing to smoulder, who can light a fuse and stand the heat. Community acupuncture needs people who are untroubled by being unimportant and glad to take care of other people who are unimportant. Community acupuncture needs people who are happy to be seen as ruffians by other acupuncturists, who can defy and shock the social norms of the acupuncture profession.

Later, she adds, "Not only are we punks, we are radicals."[8]

Deadman's reply is a reaction to both the personal criticism of acupuncturists and to the changes called for in acupuncture practice. Regarding the former, he notes, "... she has clearly worked tirelessly on behalf of financially challenged patients and practitioners," but then summarizes her critique in a tone verging on sarcasm.

> The implication and sometimes overt statement that runs through the article is that community acupuncture's way is the right, the only, way to practise. Acupuncturists who don't get it, who don't get on board, belong to the discredited "professional culture of acupuncture," yearning for respectability. They are "too well-socialised" to adopt her revolutionary model which fails to deliver the importance they crave.[9]

Rohleder's article had touched a nerve in a mainstay of the Western acupuncture profession by attacking its very identity as a profession. Like Chen Zhiqian, the architect of the Ding County experiment in 1930s China, and the striking workers from Lincoln Hospital's mental health services program in the 1960s, she held that the basic healthcare needs of the masses are best served not by professionals but by ordinary people who have undergone sufficient training in useful techniques. Her denigration of those who pursue education for education's sake, her dismissal of the reliance on sophisticated Chinese medicine theories in treatment, and her suggestion that acupuncturists should work more for less money formed a radical critique of the acupuncture education and practice that has evolved from the 1970s to the present day. She has been, indeed, the little child calling out that the emperor has no clothes.

## Working Class Acupuncture

Deadman's argument against Rohleder's model of community acupuncture contends, in essence, that it goes against best practice and therefore is not in the patient's best interest. Limiting the patient intake—the traditional 10 questions and four examinations of Chinese medicine, including observation, palpation, questioning/listening, and smelling—to the three minutes allotted by Rohleder, dispensing with pattern diagnosis (the keystone of TCM diagnosis and treatment) and eliminating the use of acupuncture points aside from those on the extremities and head were, to him, unacceptable blows to the practice of acupuncture. Rohleder's rationale for the changes was, in one sense, a simple arithmetic calculation: You cannot care for six patients an hour if you spend 45 minutes with each. On a more fundamental level, though, she was saying that spending 45 minutes per patient is a luxury that cannot be afforded by either working-class patients or working-class practitioners; community acupuncturists of Rohleder's school identify with the working class, forming a central alliance with the patients they seek.

Rohleder was educated at the Oregon College of Oriental Medicine (OCOM), considered one of the top-tier acupuncture colleges in the

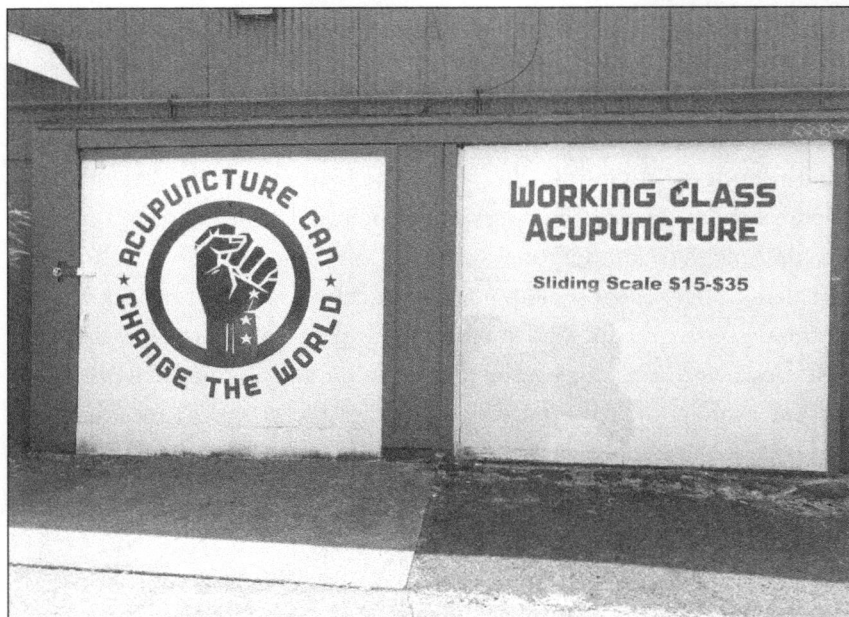

*Outside of Working Class Acupuncture's flagship location in Portland, Oregon. The stars on the wrist of the raised-fist logo indicate the Heart channel in traditional Chinese medicine. Photo by the author.*

United States. (She also holds a bachelor's degree from Bryn Mawr.) Having entered as a seeker of something yet to be defined, she seethed through most of her three-plus years there, feeling alienated from almost everything—except her partner of a lifetime Skip Van Meter, another outcast whom she met in the college clinic—until she began working shifts as an observer at an offsite clinic called Hooper Detox as part of her clinical training. The similarity to the name of the South Bronx clinic was no coincidence; the engine behind Hooper was an energetic New York transplant named David Eisen, who had worked with Michael Smith at Lincoln Detox and was a cofounder of NADA.[10] Hooper played a public health role as well, through a partnership with a local social services agency; named for David Hooper, reportedly the last person to die of alcoholism in the Portland city jail, in 1971, it served as an intervention of last resort for people caught by the police while drunk or high on heroin—rather than being jailed, they were given up to two weeks to detoxify in Hooper's residential treatment program.[11] It was at Hooper, Rohleder would later write, that she first saw acupuncture taken out of the individualized context in which she was being taught—where it was "all about the brilliance of the practitioner illuminating the uniqueness of each patient"—and replaced by daily, routine treatments, the results incrementally accruing. Patients sat in hard chairs under fluorescent lights, but they sat in a circle together, each getting essentially the same treatment, which was the form of ear acupuncture known as the NADA protocol and developed at Lincoln Detox. There were no white coats. Rohleder felt it was "low-key, humble, unthreatening."[12]

After graduating, she and Van Meter continued to work in public health programs, providing acupuncture while dabbling in private practice, renting single rooms from other healthcare practices or sometimes working out of their home. In 2002, after eight years of struggling to make a living in acupuncture while raising a family, Rohleder decided to rent a larger space where she could treat multiple people at once. The space ended up being much larger—2,000 square feet, filled with the remnants of a failed thrift store. To make it look homey, she and Van Meter populated it with reclining chairs from Goodwill and lamps resting on end tables salvaged from the thrift store debris. Over the next few years, they worked out, empirically, their model of community acupuncture. Having lost their jobs in public health acupuncture when funding dried up and having voluntarily given up the individually focused style they had learned in school, they decided to, as Rohleder likes to say, "break the binary"—the binary being either government-funded group ear acupuncture or highly priced individual treatments in spa-like private rooms. They set a sliding scale and scheduled multiple treatments per hour, making up in volume what they lacked in price. People were invited to stay in the recliners as long as they wanted. Ear acupuncture was used, but so were points on the arms and legs; points on the trunk of the body were not, as it was clearly both impractical and insensitive to ask patients relaxing in chairs within a group to remove any clothing. (Later, as the clinic adopted the concept of trauma-centered care, it also became evident that it would be inappropriate to ask people who may have been sexually traumatized to undress under any circumstances.)

Eventually, Rohleder came up with a definition of community acupuncture: acupuncture delivered in a communal setting, in such a way as to make it accessible and affordable in frequent doses to as many people as possible, while being committed to social justice in healthcare and remaining financially self-sustaining. Rohleder never strays far from the business model and the concept of social entrepreneurship in describing her clinic, but her commitment to it is deeply personal. She frequently describes herself, defiantly, as "white trash"; to her, the clinic was a place where she could provide a refuge for people like herself, where they could be "at the center instead of at the margins."[13]

The clinic, named Working Class Acupuncture, grew steadily. In 2010, it delivered 31,000 treatments; by 2018, having expanded to three sites, it provided more than 56,000.[14] WCA, as it is commonly known, provides a salary and benefits, including paid vacation, to its employees—rarities in the world of acupuncture employment, in which 88 percent of acupuncturists are self-employed.[15] If she were a typical entrepreneur, Rohleder could have sat back and been satisfied with her results; she and Van Meter were making a living and the children were grown, the clinic was reaching large numbers of Portland's working and middle classes, and it was providing a living wage to local, like-minded acupuncturists. But she was neither typical nor satisfied. The larger world—of acupuncture education, of healthcare, of social inequity—still needed changing, and Rohleder set out to change it. Within a dozen years, she launched a national nonprofit (the Community Acupuncture Network), an international cooperative (POCA), and an iconoclastic acupuncture college (POCA Tech), and published three books on her radical vision for community acupuncture as a fomenter of social change. Within the next six years, she initiated a partnership with Oregon's largest Medicaid provider, CareOregon, and defined an overarching mission for the movement through the articulation of a new philosophy, Liberation Acupuncture.

## The People's Organization of Community Acupuncture

WCA gave Rohleder the means to create a low-key, humble, and unthreatening environment—a "safe space" in the social justice lexicon—to attract the working-class patients with whom she most identified. In forming POCA, she did the same for acupuncturists. WCA was successful in part because it reached a previously unmined vein of people who might never have had an acupuncture treatment because of the expense and because it was not the type of thing they imagined themselves doing. (Lisa Achilles, who as a specialist team leader at CareOregon was a crucial link in the partnership with WCA, said of her first experience with acupuncture, "I remember thinking two things: I don't want needles because it's going to hurt and, two, I've got to be honest, this is something white people do. Black people don't do this.")[16] As it turned out, there was a similarly underground trove of disenchanted acupuncturists who had been struggling to find meaning and earn a living in a world that, until then, had seemed to be missing something vital.

The formation of POCA was announced in the third edition of *The Little Red Book of Community Acupuncture* in 2011. By this time, a growing network of sympathetic acupuncturists had emerged through the nonprofit Community Acupuncture Network, an open-source, online support group founded by Rohleder and Van Meter on the back of interest generated from her erstwhile *Acupuncture Today* column. As the number of community clinics in the United States swelled—Rohleder's figures show it jumped from 11 in 2006 to 200 in 2011[17]—it became clear the movement needed a more formal governing structure, one that would include not only acupuncturists but community acupuncture patients, clinics, and other organizations supporting POCA's mission of creating "a stable and sustainable economic foundation for the delivery of affordable acupuncture."[18] The cooperative employs a sociocratic model of governance, distinguished from a democracy or an autocracy in that it is governed by the individuals who interact within it, with decisions based on consent rather than, for example, majority rule.[19]

The Latin root "socius" has distinctly nonthreatening definitions—companion, comrade, partner, colleague, accomplice, or ally—that happen to fit perfectly with POCA's safe-space ethos. When members raise emotive topics, they tend to couch their delivery in nonalienating tones; a discussion on racism, during a gathering in Portland in June 2018, was led by two young women who began, "White people have a tendency to think of white supremacy as something outside of ourselves. We ask you to, like, sit with 'that's not true.'"[20] Even the POCA logo has taken revolution to a safer space; in contrast to WCA's logo—a raised fist in revolutionary red, contained within a circle, and surrounded by the words "Acupuncture can change the world"—POCA is represented by a fully tilted reclining chair in forest green.

The cooperative's mild-mannered mission statement is belied by the fervent dedication of its members. Underlying the benign goal of making acupuncture more affordable percolates a brew of discontent and a belief that acupuncture can indeed be employed to change the world. The gathering in Portland was headlined "Liberation Acupuncture and Community-Based Integrative Medicine"; it was advertised as a fundraiser and sponsored by CareOregon. The weekend event featured a number of panel discussions and workshops, which sometimes brought to mind collective meetings circa 1970: two people knitted; a woman nursed her baby. On the floor, an ancient dog snored loudly. There was a lot of frayed attire, worn in creative layers, and innovative body piercings. But the passion was fully in the moment. "What we're doing is trying to leverage the resources we have to be more relevant," said a woman from Seminole Heights Community Acupuncture in Florida, describing her community as one where 50 percent of five-year-old children lived in food-insecure families. She defined a punk as "a person who uses acupuncture as a tool to make a fairer world."[21] Members spoke of working with refugees and former prisoners and partnering with suboxone and methadone clinics. Another woman broke down in tears while explaining how transgender people were discriminated against in her community.

POCA gave community acupuncturists benefits that all movements share: strength in numbers and a common identity (to the extent they call the world they inhabit "the POCAverse"). It also gave them something specific with which to approach the world of conventional healthcare: an understanding of their own organizational culture. "It would be very hard to interact with another organization's culture unless you're rooted in your own," Cris Monteiro, who worked closely with Rohleder in establishing POCA, said.[22] Part of the struggle community acupuncture faces is how to reach the patients who lack the relative benefits of either the working or middle classes—those with virtually no resources of their own—and how to be compensated for caring for them. One of the thorniest dilemmas of social entrepreneurship is how to do social good while making money, and the uneasy relationship with capitalism is always on display at POCA gatherings. A case in point is the partnership between WCA and CareOregon that began in 2012; the relationship has in some ways been seminal to Rohleder's vision. Under the agreement, WCA began providing acupuncture treatments to some of CareOregon's most "difficult" clients, through a process known as hot-spotting, whereby a healthcare system identifies a subset of high-utilizing patients—the kind who turn up frequently in the emergency room. For two years, WCA offered the treatments at no cost to either the patient or CareOregon before working out a reimbursement mechanism and expanding the partnership through a pain management pilot project and a community-benefits grant program for women living in shelters. The entire program falls under the umbrella of "trauma-informed care," an approach to healthcare oriented around the pervasiveness of trauma and the avoidance of retraumatizing attitudes or actions.[23]

The partnership has been mutually beneficial in multiple ways, but least of these is the financial benefit to WCA; from the first initiative, the Health Resilience program, the clinic made less than $13,000 from 2014 to 2018, and from all three programs it grossed less than $40,000.[24]

Rohleder made a list of her clinic's return on investment from the relationship, beginning with validation of the community acupuncture vision and a sense of shared purpose with other safety-net clinicians. "It's that feedback, that what we're already doing is what people need," she said. "There is a tremendous social element to acupuncture and a huge social element to healing. People suffer from all kinds of symptoms but suffer enormously from marginalization and not being welcomed." She added, "A lot of what we got [was] validation, ironically from an insurance company, that we never got from other acupuncture clinics."[25] Most importantly, however, she found the key to articulating the philosophy that had been forming in her mind through all her years of experience with healing.

The philosophy of Liberation Acupuncture evolved as the community acupuncture movement evolved; there was no sudden revelation. Rohleder tends to perceive events and insights as coming to her in quiet or unexpected or sometimes inexplicable ways. When asked to specify what the term meant, she said, "We just got it a couple of years ago." Asked to expand on "got it," she replied, "Got it as a concept, articulated it. Liberation movements are fluid, they don't have a fixed definition." However, she said, "The arrival of trauma-informed care was key in being able to articulate what we were doing."[26] CareOregon's Health Resilience program introduced Rohleder to the concepts of trauma-informed care and led her to an analysis of the social determinants of health, which in turn clarified her thinking around the interrelating elements of health, suffering, injustice, and inequality that had been circulating in her consciousness for so long. From these ideas she was able to formulate a unifying philosophical foundation on which community acupuncture could rest.

## Liberation Acupuncture

Liberation Acupuncture harks to several historical movements and personalities. Among them are the founders of Lincoln Detox, some of whom were members and supporters of the Black liberation move-

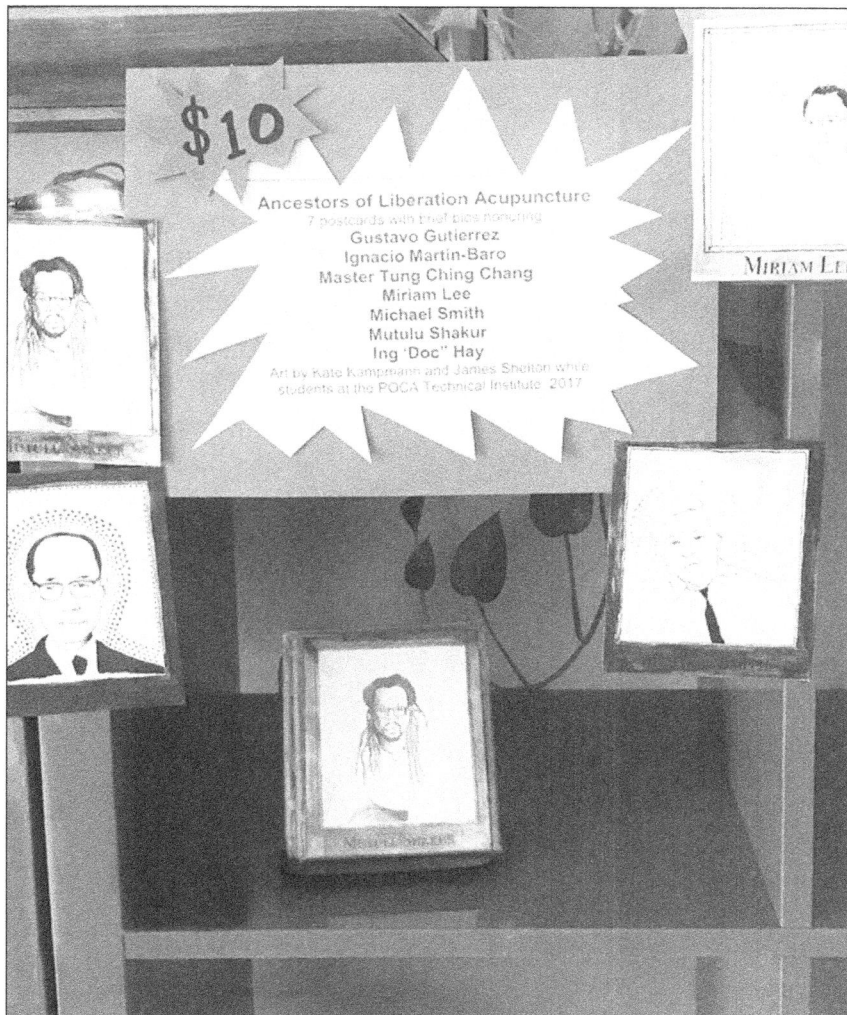

*Postcards representing "Ancestors of Liberation Acupuncture" on display at Working Class Acupuncture in Portland, Oregon. Clockwise from top right, they depict Miriam Lee, Michael Smith, Mutulu Shakur, and Master Tung. Postcards designed by Kate Kampmann and James Shelton. Photo by the author.*

ment; the founders of NADA, including Michael Smith; Miriam Lee, who was arrested in California in 1974 for practicing acupuncture; Ing "Doc" Hay, like Lee a Chinese immigrant, who suffered racist attacks while using Chinese medicine to treat the townspeople in John Day, Oregon, in the late 1800s; and the Spanish-born Jesuit priest and social psychologist Ignacio Martin-Baró, a proponent of liberation psychology who worked with peasants in El Salvador and was assassinated by the El Salvadoran army in 1989. Rohleder was drawn to these particular individuals in part because of one commonality: They all suffered for their commitment to their beliefs.

Suffering is a potent theme in Liberation Acupuncture, and suffering in solidarity with the poor, the marginalized, and victims of inequality is one of its core tenets. Rohleder, who has a nonconformist but powerful faith in Christianity, has even been criticized by her own community for her emphasis on suffering and martyrdom, following a blog post in which she referenced the Liberation Theology concept of "crucified peoples" as "those who are routinely dehumanized by violent and oppressive systems throughout history."[27] (The logo for Liberation Acupuncture is the same as that for WCA—a raised fist in dark red, with three stars on the ulnar side corresponding to points along the Heart channel as defined by TCM.)

The theoretical literature on which the movement rests bears comparison to that used by radical movements of the 1960s and 70s. Three books central to the Young Lords' intellectual education were Che Guevara's *Man and Socialism: Transformation of the Individual*; Mao Zedong's *Little Red Book*, and Frantz Fanon's *The Wretched of the Earth*.[28] Fanon's book, which as the name suggests is rife with descriptions of suffering, was widely read by activists from the BPP to the MBGC. Liberation Acupuncture has Rohleder and Van Meter's own *Little Red Book* and a handful of other treatises authored by Rohleder, the most recent of which, *Acupuncture Points Are Holes*, is subtitled *A Case Study in Social Entrepreneurship* but presents the case study through a prism of suffering.

The concept has matured into a full philosophy since then, in line with the tenets of Liberation Psychology, which "originate in critiques of psychology as individualistic and acontextual and as potentially oppressive especially through racist, sexist, ethnocentric, homophobic and class biases," and that involves "participatory practices that aim to avoid reproducing oppression" while engaging in a "critical reflection of power and privilege."[29] The description is very close to that of the radical therapy movement of the 1970s, which was employed by staff in the early days of the Lincoln Detox clinic. It is also an accurate portrayal of a typical POCAfest workshop, which may begin with a critical reflection on members' own power and privilege and continue into a discussion of how they can avoid reproducing oppression in their clinics.

Perhaps most central to Liberation Acupuncture is its understanding that "individual health and disease do not exist, and cannot be understood or addressed, apart from social conditions—particularly injustice, inequality, and the pervasive influence of traumatic stress."[30] It therefore frames its entire approach in reference to the priorities of people who have been oppressed, exploited, or traumatized by society. Rohleder's worldview has always included the community acupuncture practitioner as potentially oppressed—by the for-profit educational system, by capitalism, by the Ming vase majority. At the same time, her movement is acutely conscious of the acupuncturist's position of power and privilege in relation to her most marginalized patients. There is thus a paradoxical feeling of alliance with the oppressed and a need to atone for one's privilege—evoking shades of the philosophical and emotional dilemma the MBGC felt as white supporters of Black and brown liberation movements.

There proved a further usefulness to having a guiding philosophy. In 2014 Rohleder and Van Meter opened POCA Tech, a low-cost technical college designed to train community acupuncturists. Early deliberations with the ACAOM, which accredits all US acupuncture colleges, were sometimes difficult; ACAOM representatives indicated they were not satisfied with limits on teaching the full range of acupuncture points and theories that Deadman had criticized in the pages of the *JCM* years earlier. Rohleder is a reluctant intellectual, and, having fully articulated her philosophy to the world at large, she wrote a blog post declaring, "What we really wanted to say was that acupuncture works if it works in real life, for ordinary people, and whatever allows ordinary people to use acupuncture in a way that works for them is more valid than an academic theory that you can't/shouldn't do acupuncture like that. Apparently the way to say it so that academics can hear it is 'Liberation Acupuncture.'"[31]

## POCA Tech

POCA Tech may be the most difficult acupuncture college in the United States to get into. Most of the roughly 50 accredited colleges require certain academic credentials and some ability to pay, usually through federal financial aid, which they facilitate; POCA Tech requires applicants to read Rohleder's book, *Acupuncture Points Are Holes*. Many either withdraw their application after reading it or are rejected based on their reaction. Those who are rejected fall into one of the following categories outlined by Rohleder: "People who have an abstract vision for this. People who think the capitalist fantasy will work. Or people who are fascinated with the medium."[32] She is adamant that students who are intoxicated by the perfume of exotic theories and artifacts are not the right material for the school, whose main function is to produce more community acupuncturists to staff POCA clinics. The students who do enroll, says Rohleder, are "people who can't stand the way the world is. People who love taking care of people. People who are refugees from other parts of society."[33] In other words, they are people sympathetic to the POCAverse and to the construct of Liberation Acupuncture.

Most POCA Tech students were not primarily interested in acupuncture initially. "It wasn't because of acupuncture, but the mission," one student said of her attraction to the college. Another said she spent 17 years in social justice work before applying. When asked what made her leave social work, she paused. "Ah. That's funny. I think I finally found it." She continued, "I remember the first couple years I was telling people, especially in my field, 'You guys, you don't understand—we're actually doing it.' And everybody in my field was like, 'No.' They couldn't believe it, like, 'You figured it out.'"

Social workers may have been delighted, but the mainstream acupuncture community has been less so. In January 2018, the Acupuncture Advisory Board of Utah wrote a letter of concern to the NCCAOM, which oversees certification exams; the majority of states use the NCCAOM exams as a basis for licensure. The letter expressed dismay at what it called a request by POCA Tech to lower educational standards, a reference in part to the college's format; classes meet for one long weekend per month rather than weekly. However, the main argument was that Chinese herbology is not part of the curriculum. It was a peculiar complaint because several mainstream acupuncture colleges already offered degrees in acupuncture alone, and passing the NCCAOM exam for herbs is not a licensure requirement in some states, including Utah. The omission of herbology, the letter stated, was of deep concern to the integrity of the profession and the safety of the public. The Utah Acupuncture Licensing Board responded with a proposed rule change amendment that would essentially ban POCA Tech graduates from practicing in Utah by adding a licensure requirement to pass the NCCAOM exam in Chinese herbology.

Turf wars are not new in licensed professions, but the proposed ban would have hit the new college disproportionately; around 10 percent of its small student body was from Utah, and two of its sustaining members were POCA clinics in Salt Lake City. After a contentious two-hour meeting held in February 2018 at the Division of Occupational and Professional Licensing in Salt Lake City, the proposed amendment was dropped. But the experience left POCA members feeling more than ever that they were embattled outsiders confronting a biased and obdurate establishment. Perhaps adding to the competitive ire they were raising was POCA Tech's low tuition; the three-year program costs a total of around $17,000, compared to nearly $93,000 for a four-year master's degree at OCOM, Rohleder's alma mater. POCA Tech cites an equation in setting its fee: The cost of becoming an acupuncturist, including the education, certification, licensing, and start-up costs, should be roughly equal to the expected income in the first year to year and a half of practice. The equation is in stark contrast to the prevailing reality, in which most students will borrow more than $60,000, according to 2014 figures from ACAOM, the accrediting body.[34] A 2017 survey by the American Association of Acupuncture and Oriental Medicine, a national advocacy organization, reported that 40 percent of respondents had assumed more than $100,000 in loans, but only 16 percent earned enough to pay off the debt through a 30-year extended repayment plan.[35] A comment on Rohleder's blog post about the Utah controversy suggested POCA Tech's low tuition might offend graduates of more expensive colleges. Responding to her description of the acupuncture job market and curriculum at POCA Tech, the commenter said, "In essence, you were attacking the current and past training standards that thousands of acupuncturists have invested time, sweat, tears and much money into."[36]

While POCA Tech does not offer financial aid—tuition would have to double to cover administrative costs if it did[37]—graduates are not entirely debt-free upon leaving. They are required to commit three years to the cooperative, either working in a POCA clinic or opening a new one. The primary purpose behind the college is to provide more workers in POCA clinics, and applicants are evaluated with their suitability to this objective in mind. Underlying the practical aim, however, is also a goal to buck the system, to show students there is a different way of going about acupuncture; that they should not have to graduate with an unsustainable level of debt; and that much of the material taught in mainstream acupuncture colleges can be jettisoned—not only without compromising their ability as acupuncturists but, to the contrary, thereby focusing their capacity as healers serving marginalized people.

It is a lofty vision in a humble setting. Classes are held as part of the Rose City Park Collective, in a rambling, red brick building in Northeast Portland that also houses the social justice projects Do Good Multnomah and the International Justice Mission as well as Rose City Park United Methodist Church. POCA Tech has a long, narrow room next to the library. On a grey, drizzly July day, there were four tables where the seven students sat (two others were practicing needling) in the front of the room and several mismatched recliners in the rear. Skip Van Meter, dressed in a rumpled blue T-shirt, jeans, and black sneakers, was lecturing. Acupuncture charts and a poster of "Rohleder's Hierarchy of Acupuncture Needs"—an adaptation of psychologist Abraham Maslow's "Hierarchy of Needs," with "physical safety" at the bottom and "acupuncture theory" near the top—hung on the wall behind him, along with a calendar opened to a page featuring "Stonewall at 50: Rebellion to Liberation."[38] A door marked "exit" was blocked by a stepladder. Notably, there was a dearth of electronic devices; Van Meter used only a colored pen and the whiteboard, while a single student had an iPad, and no one looked at a smartphone. Another remarkable feature was contained in the lecture itself. The term was just finishing, and the class was completing its study of 10 different approaches to acupuncture, including those of Miriam Lee, the pioneering California acupuncturist who developed her own protocol, and Master Tung, who was a teacher of Lee in China and whose system of needling points distal to the affected limb or body part has gained popularity in the United States, in large part thanks to Lee. The final approach, about to be broached, was TCM. The chronology was educational heresy, as TCM is the mainstay of most American acupuncture colleges. Students who want to learn other theories, such as Lee's or Tung's, do so through continuing education units, generally after graduation.

Van Meter began with a brief history of Chinese medicine, explaining that by the 1800s, herbal medicine was favored in China while needling was being phased out. As a result, he said, TCM often equates the function of a point with the function of an herb and holds that each point has designated actions (which it evokes) and indications (for which it is chosen). "TCM for me is a little like having blinders on," he said. "It takes out the context. A point is where you put a needle, not where it's located on a chart." He concluded, "You've got to be really careful with the theories—all theories change. Your practice has to work, because making a living charging [only] a little bit of money is hard." Rounding out the lecture, he urged the students to consider

"What is the stuff you need to know a) to pass the boards, b) to effectively treat patients, and c) to run a clinic?"[39]

The didactic method was appealing in its simplicity and practicality and seemed to have more in common with the community-based approach at BAAANA and First World Acupuncture 40 years earlier than with the typical acupuncture college classroom today, although there is considerable variation. One of Rohleder's favored words is "praxis," emphasizing that nothing has true meaning apart from its implications in real life. While conducting a comparative analysis of different approaches during the lecture, Van Meter asked, "What would be the proof of concept of what works best?" His answer was praxis—that practice trumps all, and the proof is that the patient improves and comes back.[40] Most acupuncturists would argue that is their objective as well, but POCA Tech's unique approach is to strip away all but the essentials, laying bare the acupuncturist's raw desire to make a meaningful change in a hurtful world with only a handful of silver needles.

Such minimalization does not constitute a rejection of acupuncture theory. POCA Tech sees TCM as one of the less important branches of acupuncture training due to its emphasis on esoteric theories. However, the community acupuncturists do not privilege their own improvisational and experiential knowledge; they embrace a number of different techniques and systems, including those of Dr. Tung, Miriam Lee, and Richard Tan, that are based in Chinese principles of acupuncture. The systems are promulgated by eminent acupuncturists and used throughout the United States. The difference in theoretical training goes back to POCA Tech's goal to train competent, safe, and efficient acupuncturists to perform community acupuncture at an affordable price. As the only US acupuncture college to offer a certificate rather than a master's degree, they choose to see acupuncture as a trade rather than a theoretic course of study.

For Rohleder, the purpose again returned to Liberation Acupuncture. "Liberation Acupuncture gave us permission to structure the school around the needs of community acupuncture patients—which was otherwise unjustifiable academically, at least according to our early inter-actions with ACAOM [the accrediting body]," she wrote in a POCA website blog. "Liberation Acupuncture was the theory that freed us from all the other theories that claimed we shouldn't be allowed to do what we were doing, because we were devaluing acupuncture itself. Liberation Acupuncture freed us from the imaginary hierarchies and let us be truthful about the horizontal epistemology, otherwise expressed as, *there is not now and never has been one right way to do acupuncture.*"[41] [Emphasis in original]

## The Orientalization of American Acupuncture

In early 2010, well before the formation of POCA Tech, Rohleder struck up a relationship that would profoundly influence its progression. Tyler Phan is a social anthropologist who earned his PhD at University College London; he is also a Vietnamese American who comes from a distinct line of acupuncturists and who trained formally at an acupuncture college in North Carolina. In Phan, Rohleder found an intellectual partner; the two met in Frederick, Maryland, where she and Van Meter were leading a Community Acupuncture workshop. "I was up in front of the room complaining about the acupuncture profession and I mentioned everybody using bamboo in their logos," Rohleder said, "and Tyler raised his hand and said, 'The word for what you're describing is Orientalism,' and we've pretty much been friends ever since."[42] Phan's subsequent research would give academic rigor and an evidence base to her own perceptions of American acupuncture education, including the mandatory study of seemingly arbitrary subjects, the high cost-debt load, and the balance of power among accrediting and licensing agencies, individuals, and the schools themselves.

Phan began speaking at POCA gatherings, called POCAfests, describing his theories and preliminary findings. He completed his dissertation in 2017. Titled simply "American Chinese Medicine," it is an ethnography that examines power structures within academic and professional realms. The paper contends that what is currently called acupuncture in the United States is a professionalized distortion of the varied traditions brought to the country by Asian immigrants, created and promulgated by a succession of individuals who were mainly white and mainly men and who viewed the medicine through a necessarily biased cultural lens. Ultimately, the process marginalized the cultures to whom the medicine originally belonged, Phan asserts. He argues that American Chinese medicine is a product of what he calls orientalized biopower—"the process where America's predominately white counter-culture began to encompass an orientalism which romanticized a form of Chinese medicine constructed in the 1950s by the People's Republic of China called Traditional Chinese medicine (TCM)."[43]

The term is a melding of Edward Said's Orientalism and Michel Foucault's biopower. Both concepts, developed in the 1970s, deal with the themes of power, governance, and control. Orientalism is a perspective on world history that views the imbalance of power between the colonized "Orient" and the colonialist "Occident" as a result of the West's ability, first to define the East, and second to define it as "other" and therefore lesser to the West in a multitude of cultural and behavioral ways. In developing the concept of biopower, Foucault wrote of an evolution of two related forms of power: The first focused on the individual body; the second on what Foucault termed "the species body, the body imbued with the mechanics of life and serving as the basis of the biological processes." During the evolution of these forms of power, from the seventeenth to the eighteenth centuries, there was, Foucault wrote, "an explosion of numerous and diverse techniques for achieving the subjugation of bodies and the control of populations, marking the beginning of an era of 'biopower.'"[44]

Phan tells a narrative of seven white researchers at UCLA in the mid-1970s, which he calls the UCLA cohort. Like the radical medical interns and doctors at Lincoln Hospital, they were active in the anti-Vietnam movement and other left-wing protests, and they became interested in tai chi and, subsequently, acupuncture. In 1971, shortly after Reston's article on acupuncture was published in the *New York Times*, they formed the National Acupuncture Association, which became a research group through their affiliation with UCLA's medical school.[45] In 1972, they worked with a California legislator to pass AB-1500, mandating that acupuncture could only be practiced by unlicensed individuals if they were within "an approved medical school for the primary purpose of scientific investigation" and under the supervision of a licensed medical doctor.[46] However, there were no state acupuncture licenses and, as Phan points out, the new law was then joined with an existing clause in California's business and professional code to prosecute Asian practitioners of Chinese medicine whose knowledge and practice predated the revelations about acupuncture among the UCLA cohort and their ilk.

By the end of the decade, members of the cohort had helped in the formation of colleges on the East and West coasts, including the New England School of Acupuncture in Massachusetts, where Ted Kaptchuk would teach before moving on to Harvard Medical School. They were also involved in establishing licensing boards, professional lobbying organizations, and curricula in various states, including California, Nevada, New York, and Oregon. Phan describes their motivation as "a desire to professionalize and, in most cases, follow in the footsteps of the American Medical Association."[47]

Phan creates a subcategory of Orientalism to encompass the UCLA cohort and its impact on American Chinese medicine: counterculture Orientalism, borne of the disaffected—and again, predominantly white and male—well-educated youth of the 1960s-70s era. This group, searching for new identities after rejecting the ones they were raised with, romanticized Eastern culture without being sensitive to anti-Asian discrimination—or, at worst, being complicit in it. He argues it is this brand of Orientalism that "would shape the gaze and construction of American Chinese medicine."[48]

"The gaze," Phan explained at a POCAfest workshop in Toronto in 2018, is "the way you view the medicine, and the bodies, the ideas, and the practices." The underlying problem, as he sees it, is that the UCLA cohort took power of the gaze and in that way took control of the medicine from those who were now only subjects of the gaze. He condensed his thesis: "My whole dissertation's point is to say that these professions are built on a house of cards—there's nothing substantial about these laws … none of it's empirically based." Referring to the disparate lineages of Chinese medicine, he said, "They're trying to standardize what a Chinese medicine is. And create the standards for the profession. This is highly dangerous! Because not only is it based on a house of cards—nothing—but it also will create marginalization."

In fact, Phan goes further than warning of marginalization; he sees "institutional, systematic white supremacy" in American Chinese medicine.

> In anything with medicine, you have to look into the context of the knowledge production. Who teaches you to do Chinese medicine? Well in the United States, it is predominantly white. And it's predominantly men … So that creates this interesting dynamic in itself, of who controls the medicine, literally who controls it, so the domination and the superiority of white supremacy is in the actual governance of the medicine itself. It's hugely problematic.

Putting his themes into layman's language, Phan attempted an extended metaphor of the most American thing he could think of: apple pie. The educational framework offers three basic kinds of pie, he said: Sara Lee—"It's very manufactured, same ingredients, same product, price may fluctuate a little bit, but it tastes the same"; an overpriced artisanal pie—"It's, I don't know, $800 for a workshop to learn this kind of method"; and the pie baked from a recipe passed from generation to generation, which he likened to the carefully guarded family lineages of acupuncture, not available in stores or acupuncture colleges. Someone asked what kind of pie POCA produces. He thought for a moment. "POCA gets a lot of the good stuff from familial lineages and some mass-produced stuff," he said. "So I'm thinking it's kind of like the Costco, it's like the familial stuff but like Costco—good prices, you get insane stuff, you get it in bulk, you know what I mean?" He added, "I love Costco. I'm a huge Costco fan."[49]

In December 2019, POCA Tech momentarily announced plans to open a campus in Pittsburgh, Pennsylvania, with Phan at the helm. While the plan was withdrawn a few weeks later due to logistical difficulties, expansion remains a goal—and Phan's statement in the press release remains a guiding principle. The statement began, "Healthcare is a human right, but who will provide it?" It continued, "People are in pain everywhere in this country with limited access to proper care. From rural America to underserved cities, there is a national shortage of quality healthcare providers. We have a solution, community acupuncture." The statement concluded, "With your help, we can directly impact the future of healthcare in this country by supporting a vision of liberation and service."[50] From an historical perspective, it neatly linked the theme of healthcare as a human right, which was central to the vision and practice of revolutionary detox acupuncture and First World Acupuncture, with the concept of liberation. That in turn was a core element of 1970s activism, encompassing everything from radical therapy and freedom from drug addiction to the Black liberation and Puerto Rican independence movements. The question remains of how far the revolutionary vision can go. The undercurrent of violence, whether activist or state sponsored, that troubled the former movement is gone. POCA nonetheless contends with "structural violence" (an example of structural violence is the impenetrability of bureaucracy). To date, Rohleder's vision has been fueled by an edge of anger against the norms of society and particularly against the norms of American acupuncture education. Can she construct an educational revolution from the inside out? POCA appears geared up for the fight, although in typical reclining-chair revolution fashion, the call to arms is simply, "to get community acupuncture to more places and people who need it."[51]

# CHAPTER 6

# What Now?
# The Revolution's Legacy

I f the story of revolutionary acupuncture were purely historical, one might assess its success or failure in the context of its time. If that assessment had taken place a decade or two ago, it might have arrived at a different conclusion than today. As things stand, there is a general resurgence of interest in the era in which it began, as seen in academic works, documentaries, and popular entertainment, such as the film *The Trial of the Chicago Seven* and the miniseries *Who Killed Malcolm X?*—both of which aired on Netflix in 2020. In the face of Black Lives Matter and the struggle against the values and policies surrounding the era of Donald Trump, even 1970s-era movements are seeing a chance for renaissance, as when the radical science movement Science for the People, which lasted from 1969 to 1989, began a revival in 2015 (it is also the subject of a recent scholarly book, *Science for the People: Documents from America's Movement of Radical Scientists*).[1] There is a new urgency to our collective memories of the time, along with reinterpretations of their meaning, as it becomes clear that many of the era's critical problems—such as drug addiction, environmental devastation, racial injustice, mass incarceration, and US military aggression—are very much alive today. At the same time, among progressive sectors there is a newfound appreciation for the radicalism of the past, which is not mired in previous perceptions of dangerous militancy or counter-cultural weirdness.

Radical movements of the 1960s and 70s generally proved unsustainable, although each fell apart for specific reasons (Science for the People held together for an atypically long time and ultimately was undone by back taxes).[2] Factionalism and infiltration from the FBI were common factors that affected organizations including the Black Panthers and the Young Lords as well as the revolutionaries at BAAANA. Ironically, Joanna Fernández describes the lumpenproletariat—the most oppressed class of society, including street people and drug addicts, who were courted to some extent by radical groups as those most suited to lead the revolution—as a factor in the revolution's downfall. The lumpen's susceptibility to FBI recruitment created a weak link in the BPP and the Young Lords that the groups' internal structure could not rectify, Fernández contends.[3] This was arguably a weakness at BAAANA as well, based on Bayau Kamete's actions, although BAAANA's calamitous downfall was a direct result of the Brink's "expropriation" and drug use and indirectly a consequence of some members' involvement in other militant actions. While the seriousness of using lethal force cannot be mitigated, the motivation can be understood as complex. In the context of relentless racial oppression and extrajudicial killings of African Americans, revolutionaries saw themselves in a state of war against the government and were "tired of seeing all the bodies just on one side."[4]

In terms of social and political revolution, the movement was unable to achieve its goals. Recently, historians have shed insight into the failure of larger US revolutionary organizations of the 1960s and 70s to meet their world-changing aspirations. In particular, the inability to attract a mass following limited their potential for meaningful, broad-based social change.[5] Beyond these limitations, though, the actions at BAAANA culminating in the Brink's episode were an unquestionably fatal blow to revolutionary detox acupuncture. Even radical left activists disavowed it; as Susan Reverby writes, in her biography of Barbara Zeller's husband Alan Berkman, "Very few were willing to support the claims that this was political action by enemy combatants in a war the United States was raging against black militancy."[6] Yet the situation was complicated for revolutionary detox acupuncture. Not everyone at BAAANA was aware of its connection to militant liberation groups. Even most May 19th members were not apprised of the underground actions that led to the Brink's catastrophe.[7] Somehow healing and violence, drug detoxification and drug use, became tangled up in the increasingly chaotic milieu of revolutionary politics, liberation militancy, and violent state-sponsored repression. The result has had lasting repercussions on this chapter in the history of North American acupuncture. Unfortunately, it has obscured the valuable contributions of Black, Latinx, and other left activists to a lineage of social justice healing that is gaining prominence today.

The legacy of criminal indictment still hangs heavily over the history of BAAANA. Most notably, Mutulu Shakur remains in prison, where at the age of 70 he has survived a stroke and COVID-19 and has been treated since late 2019 for advanced cancer. His legal team's petitions for compassionate release have nonetheless been rejected, raising another significant topic of injustice: the harsh treatment of the aging population in the US prison system.[8] Shakur, who is the stepfather of the late rapper Tupac, has continued while in prison to promote social justice, including advocating for a truth and reconciliation commission in the United States, which he frames in the context of the history of slavery, segregation, racism, and the fight for civil rights.[9]

Shakur's supporters, especially those who were with him at BAAANA, have been reluctant to speak of its history, in part out of sensitivity to his legal situation, in part due to a lingering fear of the FBI. For these reasons, and because of the persistent disaffection for the Brink's action, the history of revolutionary detox acupuncture has until recently been confined to the memories of a few. Instead, the history of acudetox was identified with the development of NADA at Lincoln Detox by Michael Smith after the revolutionaries were removed. The broader history of radical movements of the 1960s and 70s is being reevaluated, however, and contemporary voices for radical change are rising in the fields of integrative medicine and acupuncture, creating possibilities for a more sympathetic understanding of this flawed but important history.

The preceding chapters have described three revolutionary movements in acupuncture; however, "revolution" took on different forms and meanings in each. Revolutionary detox acupuncture was borne in the context of the revolutionary politics of the 1960s and early 70s, a time when New Left politics were informed by Third World Marxism and militancy was a common tactic. First World Acupuncture sought a balance between two eras: It tried to maintain the spirit and vision of its predecessor but without the strident rhetoric or underground actions. What made First World Acupuncture truly revolutionary was its re-envisioning of acupuncture education and provision. It was a foundational model of a North American acupuncture college created to train primarily Black and Latinx people to serve their communities. It was the first college to proclaim service to the community as its mission and vision while offering a degree specifically to this end. Its clinic put the vision into action, offering acupuncture to people in need of low-cost, low-tech healing—especially those with health problems stemming from systemic socioeconomic or racial inequalities.

In this sense the clinic became a predecessor to the "offsite" clinics of many subsequent acupuncture colleges, which serve populations in need in their local areas. These clinics serve multiple purposes: They provide valuable healthcare, free at the point of service, to underserved populations; they give the college an opportunity to develop a relationship with, and reputation within, the community; and they provide a training ground for the college's interns, while exposing them to a need and a possibility for acupuncture that they may not otherwise have been made aware of through their education. Yet these clinics remain largely peripheral to the ethos of most mainstream acupuncture colleges in the United States.[10] Only POCA Tech has made service to the community its raison d'être.

Like First World Acupuncture, Liberation Acupuncture is revolutionary in its promulgation of education and acupuncture clinical care for the explicit purpose of serving communities in need. Its revolutionary mission takes place in a far different context than that of its predecessor, though, which was situated in opposition to the power of the state. That power was manifested in two major ways: First, the State of New York controlled the regulation of acupuncture (at a time when there was no pathway to licensing for First World graduates); and second, the Joint Terrorist Task Force was a continuing force of intimidation for First World associates who had been involved with liberation movements at BAAANA.

In contrast, in the early decades of the twenty-first century, POCA has situated itself in opposition to the mainstream acupuncture profession—namely, the status quo of acupuncture education, acupuncture regulation, and acupuncture practice in the United States—even as it must work with regulatory bodies for accreditation of its own college as it seeks to establish a new model for education and practice.[11] In that sense, the future of revolutionary acupuncture must lie in its ability to unsettle the tectonic plate of bureaucracy. Clearly, this is a different mission than battling state power in the 1970s.

While the revolution in these three examples has been acted out in different ways and embodied different meanings, all three movements have shared significant elements. Each has been motivated by an acute perception of the suffering of others and a desire to alleviate it. Each has named liberation as a key to ending suffering. And each has seen their actions as a manifestation of love for the common people, whether lumpenproletariat or working class. Further, their unique bond is the belief that the alleviation of emotional, physical, and societal suffering can be enacted through acupuncture.

The revolutionary history, scientization, and easy practical applicability of acupuncture have all favored its use towards these ends, such that no single definition of acupuncture can explain its unique appropriateness to the purpose. As recounted in the previous chapters, the allure of the barefoot doctor image coupled with the model's success in

China and Africa as a means for bringing healthcare to the rural poor; the use by Mao's government of acupuncture anesthesia and auricular acupuncture as political tools; the publication of scientific articles in the Western world on acupuncture's success in treating addiction and pain; and the adaptability of techniques, ranging from empirical placement of needles in the ear, to classical full-body acupuncture, to systems of needling distal body parts in a community acupuncture setting, all played a part in the adoption of acupuncture as a means of revolution. Its use as a means to end suffering, though, was felt on a more personal level by the individuals who adopted it.

## Suffering and Love

As there were differing degrees of belief in revolution at BAAANA, so were there different motivations. Some individuals had suffered the moral outrage, psychic degradation, and physical danger of oppression personally, while others had grown up in relative comfort but identified with the suffering of others. Yet, however it is experienced, the element of suffering underlies a burning demand for change; for those who have suffered in a prolonged or grievous way, those with extraordinary empathy, or those whose powers of observation are acute in absorbing and calculating the equation of harm done to beings with whom they identify, the factor of suffering may become an unbearable wrong that they must, as moral human beings, act to rectify. Susan Rosenberg writes in her memoir, *An American Radical*, of how, in spite of her middle-class upbringing, she felt tormented into action by the oppression of others, especially as a child of the 1960s exposed to daily television coverage of Vietnam War atrocities.[12]

Jackie Haught's flirtation with revolution did not last—she said she was "never angry enough"—but the search that led her to it persisted. Seeking a way to alleviate suffering, she perceives that she has evolved in her approach from revolution to Buddhism.

I have tried to understand suffering my whole life. It started out with understanding society and nature. And I saw that people were alienated from nature, that the society was so corrupt—so I became a hippie ... Because the hippie movement really was trying to build a different society. They were sophisticated revolutionaries, a lot of them—people went to live in a different world ... after that happened, what I saw clearly was that that wasn't the answer. And so the next thing I did was I kind of got into revolutionary stuff, because I saw that the society we lived in was a lot of the issue. For the suffering, needless suffering ... And then through revolution I got into acupuncture, because that's actual pain and suffering. And acupuncture works with suffering, because it is holistic. And then I worked with AIDS, and because of all those years with acupuncture and AIDS I found Buddhism. It's like an onion. I'm understanding the complexity of suffering ... There's always going to be suffering. But it can be worked with to be much less."[13]

Haught offers a counterpoint to the righteous anger entailed in the fight for change. "I never had a doubt in my mind that Mutulu [Shakur] did what he did out of love for people," she said. "All people, but particularly poor people. [People] of color but white poor people too. I never had a doubt. He has a very big heart."[14] She is not alone in placing love as an impetus behind the revolutionary acupuncture programs. Tatsuo Hirano stated it plainly: "This is why we're all there, for the love of people." Describing group clinic sessions at Lincoln, he said, "There was so much love ... There was kindness. There was sense of community, the sense of being with the people. [It was] entirely different from any hospital or clinic, [here] where people actually cared about you." Hirano's description of Shakur echoes Haught's: "Mutulu Shakur had one of the biggest hearts that I know. His love was immense ... And you felt that. 'Come here, let's get out of this drug place, let me help you.'"[15]

# Taking the Hit

For Lisa Rohleder, the matter of suffering is profound and personal. In *Acupuncture Points Are Holes*, she writes frankly about her experience growing up with poverty and sexual abuse and of her struggles with suicidal impulses as a young adult. She abandoned early plans to go to medical school and instead began working with the most marginalized populations: people dying from AIDS, destitution, and drug addiction. Her early years in acupuncture were spent in public health settings where she surrounded herself with other people's pain even while grappling with her own. While she credits daily meditation with her survival through this time, her rage against the agony of the world did not diminish.

However, she also found comfort in her religious faith—she says belief is beside the point because she cannot conceive of a godless existence—and in the philosophies of Gustavo Gutiérrez and Ignacio Martin-Baró, both Catholic priests who dedicated their lives to advocating for the poor. Both were also well acquainted with suffering. Gutiérrez, from Peru, is half Hispanic and half Indigenous, and his activity was restricted due to a painful bone condition as an adolescent; he is a founder of liberation theology, which focuses moral thought and action on understanding the reality of the poor. Gutiérrez's standing was threatened by the Catholic church after the Holy See denounced liberation theology, for its incorporation of Marxism, in 1984. Martin-Baró, a Spaniard who spent most of his working life in El Salvador, was a key figure in the formation of liberation psychology, which emphasizes the inseparability of individual health from sociopolitical circumstance; he was murdered by the Salvadoran Army in 1989.

Rohleder's perspective on suffering is multifaceted. One facet is her identification with people who are the marginalized and disregarded, the ones she wants to reach through community acupuncture. Another is her alliance with the martyrdom of the predecessors of Liberation Acupuncture, including Gutiérrez and Martin-Baró, along with the revolutionary detox acupuncturists of the 1970s and Asian-immigrant acupuncturists who were targets of discrimination. Yet another aspect is her belief that community acupuncturists should make sacrifices. She wrote, in a blog post on Liberation Acupuncture's website, "The gospel stories which culminate in the crucifixion and ultimately the resurrection of Jesus represent solidarity with and redemption of a crucified or dehumanized people." She added that, as a Christian, "I cannot separate Liberation Acupuncture from the cross." For Rohleder, that means "the point of Liberation Acupuncture is to take the hit, to suffer in solidarity with suffering people." By taking the hit, she explained, she meant that community acupuncturists should absorb some uncertainty, risk, overwork, and underpayment in pursuit of the precarious balance of socialist ideals against a capitalist economy. She views that as a practical necessity. However, she also sees a moral imperative in taking the hit, and in training the next generation of community acupuncturists to understand the imperative. In the blog, she wrote,

> We received the vision of community acupuncture from marginalized people who paid a great price for it. To take what they gave and to refuse to reciprocate the risk and the commitment is, from the kindest perspective, ungrateful, and from a less kind perspective, theft. Individual practitioners are going to do what they feel like doing (and how), but the school has a responsibility. It's a kind of mutualism: being willing to pay a price ourselves, in the same way that the people who gave us community acupuncture paid a price.[16]

Outside of POCA, individual acupuncturists dedicated to social change have taken the hit in their own way—as a moral imperative or as the only option. A large percentage of the small number who graduated from BAAANA and First World Acupuncture has dedicated their professional lives to providing healthcare to underserved communities, most of them through acupuncture. Few have chased fortune or celebrity. As one of them put it, acupuncture used for social justice is "in the ground, in the dirt, in the 'let's do this'"—not "like some of the other folks who are making quite a lot of money from acupuncture. It has nothing to do with social justice at that point." Kokayi Patterson, who met Shakur in 1972, later started the African Wholistic Health Association and was a founding member of the Acupuncture Detox Specialists Collective in Washington, DC. Having overcome addiction himself, Patterson focused his energy on combating the hold of drugs on Black communities and the roots of drug addiction in extreme poverty. Somewhat like Rohleder, Patterson exhorts acupuncturists, specifically those who are African American, to "take the hit" by providing free treatment to those without means. He described this as a "foundational pillar" for Black acupuncturists and perhaps the most important message that came from his training in New York in the 1970s.

> I think the major thing that Dr. Shakur wanted us to do … is to make sure that the least of us—not those who could afford even a sliding scale, not the middle class, not the working class, but those individuals who had no money, those individuals [are taken care of]—because that's what we did at Lincoln … because if we're talking about a liberation, and if we're talking about revolution, we have to go and deal with those individuals who have been affected the most.[17]

Not everyone agrees with the value of taking the hit. Indeed, it may be the most common criticism leveled at POCA by other acupuncturists. In one of my classes, a student remarked that "you have to practically take a vow of poverty to join them." Even Tatsuo Hirano voiced a similar opinion, telling me, "[Their] way does not build the wealth of the people. It just provides services that's doomed to hardship and poverty."[18] Hirano was referring to poverty for both the practitioners and their clients; his broader point was that acupuncture alone is not sufficient to lift communities out of deprivation and that anyone laying claim to revolution must be prepared to go beyond acupuncture.

Certainly, the revolutionary detox acupuncturists were always clear that acupuncture was only one part of their formula; political education was equally important. That approach would not be appropriate for POCA for multiple reasons, among them the diversity of their clientele, who are primarily white and unlikely to be united around a political viewpoint. However, Rohleder's appeal to suffer with the masses seems based on a similar purpose: to identify with the predicament of those you wish to help. The paradox—by Hirano's assessment—is that in so doing she is driving community acupuncturists into that predicament rather than pulling the sufferers out of it.

What would success for revolutionary acupuncture look like, then? A more inclusive and affordable brand, with people of all colors and genders having access to acupuncture education and treatment? Or does it require a fundamentally different motivation, one promoting not only a more equitable profession but a more equal society? My own experience as an educator and administrator at Pacific College of Health and Science—the largest US acupuncture school—tells me there appears to be some progress towards the former. Students at acupuncture colleges have been vociferous in demanding, in the lexicon of the moment, more equity, diversity, and inclusion in their education since the watershed murder of George Floyd by police in May 2020. It remains to be seen if the demands represent a pivotal event. I do see progress towards a critical mass of individuals moved by the force of current events, and a deeper knowledge of alternative histories of North American acupuncture, who can create a discernable shift in the profession towards equity, diversity, and inclusion.

Of course such a shift is not a revolution. While there are other organizations using acupuncture to promote social justice, such as AWB and NADA, POCA is the only one that can be described as a movement. Its philosophy (as embodied in "taking the hit") and modus operandi (community acupuncture) create natural limitations to its potential for spread. It has, however, achieved a strong measure of interest from academia, from anthropology to medical history to the study of cooperative social and economic practices. While community acupuncturists continue to do their healing work "in the dirt," they may also create broader waves of influence.

There is another branch of legacy from revolutionary detox acupuncture. For the reasons cited above following the collapse of BAAANA, Shakur's work has not been widely known among people of any color. However, more than 40 years after BAAANA was formed, there are individual acupuncturists who take daily inspiration from it. These are people who have not been part of a movement but who have come across, in various ways, some of the history of Shakur's vision for acupuncture. Some are old enough to remember the radical spirit of the era, but others were not yet born when BAAANA was formed. They find the ethos of revolutionary acupuncture highly relevant today in a world damaged by persistent racism. Moreover, there are few Black or Latinx acupuncturists in the United States, while the majority of acupuncture patients are white.

Below, four contemporary acupuncturists of different backgrounds describe their introduction to Shakur's history of revolutionary acupuncture, how it inspired them, and how it informs their practice today. One (Yvonne Scarlett) was my classmate while we were studying for our master's degrees in TCM; the others were students in my classes in the doctoral program at the Pacific College of Health and Science. One of them, Tenisha Dandridge, is also an activist historian of revolutionary acupuncture and a collaborator with me on a conference presentation on the subject. While we rarely discussed the issue of race in class, it was clear through these women's writings that being Black in America strongly influenced their perspective on acupuncture, health, and healing. It was also evident they knew something of Mutulu Shakur's use of acupuncture. As I was researching and writing this book, I was intrigued to find what they knew of Shakur, how they understood it, and how they incorporated it into their own lives.

## A Friend of Marcus Books

Felicia Parker-Rodgers grew up in the Bay Area of San Francisco in the 1960s and 70s. After more than two decades as a licensed clinical social worker (LCSW), she practices acupuncture in North Carolina. Parker-Rodgers discovered acupuncture through a former classmate who studied it and through her aunt, a political activist who had friends who were acupuncturists. However, her introduction to radical healthcare and to Shakur came when she was a child. As preadolescents, she and her brother attended summer programs at Marcus Books, the oldest African American bookstore in the United States. Owned and operated by the Richardson family since 1960, Marcus Books has been a center of Black culture, literature, music, and political discussion, hosting the likes of James Baldwin, Malcolm X, Rosa Parks, and Toni Morrison at locations in San Francisco and Oakland.[19] As Parker-Rodgers recalls, Shakur was "a friend of Marcus Books," and he was among many Black political or cultural icons whose portraits were framed in the bookstore and whom the children learned about.

> Myself and my brother were involved in a "Rights of Passage" program. We would meet at the bookstore where there were other kids. We learned poems, songs, history, cooking, collective work, sewing, making medicine with herbs and grinding them, gardening, tilling dirt and working together as kids with adults … The bookstore had an upstairs and downstairs; downstairs was where we met. There were comfortable sofas, chairs, cushions, round tables for activities and lots of growing, leafy plants in now what I know to be clay pots. Clay pots were painting activities that we completed to add to what was already there. We were kids arriving in the late mornings and stayed for some time. I remember there was a toaster, blender, tea bags and cups, and incense burning. There was a room in the back that had a long African print curtain; adults would be in this location.
>
> I never met [Shakur] but remember there was a picture of him and many others. There were lots of framed pictures everywhere of people that we had to learn about … We had a field trip to a farm and to various farmers' markets and [learned

about] using herbs as a first line for health and healing. [There were] a lot of visitors from Nigeria and others from Africa.

Dr. Mutulu informs my practice each day. Dr. Mutulu's message asks that we examine alternative health methods, support social justice and help those who are often on the front line as political conduits. By training I am an LCSW and BCD [Board Certified Diplomate in Clinical Social Work] now for some 22-plus years, and I realize the importance of helping others to empower themselves to conserve or retain their health.[20]

## "Do You Speak Chinese?"

Yvonne Scarlett was born in Jamaica and raised her family in New York City before moving to Florida to study acupuncture. She is currently an acupuncturist in Southern California, where she combines a private practice with working shifts at a publicly funded clinic for low-income patients, a program she was instrumental in creating. The demand at the clinic can be overwhelming, but the work is important to Scarlett's sense of purpose.

My aim and agenda is to bring TCM to the majority—not as a medicine of last resort, but as primarily preventive, and second for the treatment of common diseases and concerns—for anything and everything, except trauma cases. My aim is to treat lots of women and children. Introducing this medicine to children hopefully will create a shift in the next generation who will utilize TCM and other holistic modalities first, for preventive medicine to keep serious illness and disease at bay. I serendipitously came to TCM through a series of health challenges as a last resort. The medicine was so powerful in treating several health concerns that I wanted to bring the knowledge of this medicine to people like me—people who had no idea of other holistic options for care—educated Black people, people who had given their power to the medical doctors.

I had heard of Mr. Shakur from one of my classmates, a woman of color, while I was in attendance at Florida College of Integrative Medicine, in Orlando, Florida. My recollection is that he had either started the program in New York City, and/or was involved in providing treatments to an underserved population ... I was pleasantly surprised to hear of Mr. Shakur's involvement, and also disappointed that this information was never mentioned in any of the classes, even with the discussion of [James] Reston [the *New York Times* journalist] during the time of Nixon's visit to China. It was never mentioned that he, Shakur, played a role in using acupuncture for drug detox in New York City, or that he brought acupuncture to the Black communities of New York City. Based on the patient population I typically see in the clinic, that information and history may not have been transmitted, because very few "African Americans," or Blacks, or people of color, make up the current patient population.

Most people are surprised to see a Black woman in the clinic as their Chinese Medicine physician and acupuncturist. I'm often asked if I studied in China or if I speak Chinese. I've also seen the same reaction from an Asian clinician of TCM when we were introduced, as she questioned in disbelief that I was a fellow practitioner. The fact that most people of color have neither heard of, nor have been exposed to TCM and acupuncture, even among those who are affluent and educated, is disheartening.[21]

## "I'm Not Going to Be Quiet about It"

Tenisha Dandridge is a born activist. She is also a licensed acupuncturist of more than 10 years in Sacramento, California, where she runs a mobile clinic. Dandridge is perhaps the most vocal, and energetic, proponent of racial justice through acupuncture today. She is involved with numerous projects and works with a nonprofit called Designing Justice and Designing Spaces, which aims to end mass incarceration and structural inequity through innovative building design. Among her projects is a website, blackacupuncturist.com, created "in the spirit of BAAANA ... to come, to gather, and to grow for the betterment of black and brown people." She also hosts weekly online "meet and greet" sessions in which she interviews Black acupuncturists, with the proceeds originally going to support Mutulu Shakur's appeal for freedom. Dandridge heard of Shakur's involvement in acupuncture while attending a POCAfest session led by Tyler Phan. Afterwards, she began her own investigation.

> I did some research and shared this version of history and began arguing with people—"Michael Smith did not invent this history, you're altering history and I'm not going to be quiet about it."
>
> There are pockets of us trying to do social restorative justice but it's the sustainability [that is the limiting factor], so we're trying to do better this time around. We want to keep prices low but not necessarily free. I currently work with Designing Justice and Designing Spaces—the idea is to take medicine away from white spaces and give it to melanated bodies. They made pop-ups and pay practitioners to show up. I would travel from Sacramento to Oakland because there's a very different level of acceptance [in Oakland] because of Dr. [Tolbert] Small. I have needles, I will travel. Iatrophobia is real and medical trauma is real and so it is really, really hard to get melanated bodies to acupuncture. So I do the work where I can. I work in drug treatment centers and that is best way I can participate.

Dandridge describes her Chinese medicine education as excellent but is critical of the inherent racism in acupuncture colleges she felt as a student. She is dubious that racism will change soon, even with widening emphasis on racial inclusivity in the wake of George Floyd's killing in 2020 and the subsequent demonstrations against police brutality and anti-Black racism.

> [As a student] I learned a lot and felt competent and confident—it was a lot in a short period of time. There was access to so many clinical opportunities, it was off the wall. The issue … was the enormous amount of racial battle fatigue. I had a number of racial experiences. I went from an HBCU [Historically Black College and University] to a non-melanated situation and I was perpetually exposed to this and the teachers were like, "Why are you so angry?" It just continued from there, like, "I can't show this point on you because you're too dark," or people who feel really comfortable using "that" word, because they had a Black friend, child, whatever. It was really insane the number of times I'd go through this. A friend of mine cracked a slave joke. I'm like, "You are being unleashed on the population as a healer!"
>
> Ten years later [the college] is the same. Acupuncture schools are the same, with the exception of maybe POCA Tech. This is not new, this is not news, this is politics. I think when the dust is settled, we'll all go back to status quo. I think that everyone will put together a class or two or three and then they'll fall by the wayside.[22]

## Informed by Black Militancy Movements

Like Felicia Parker-Rodgers, Monica Garcia grew up in the Bay Area—San Francisco—although in a different era. Yet while she was raised in the 1980s and 90s, she also had a strong sense of the political figures of earlier times; inspired by the adults around her, including a high school teacher and her mother, who drove her to bookstores, she read works such as *The Autobiography of Malcolm X* and Frantz Fanon's *Black Skin, White Masks*. She was also a fan of Tupac Shakur and read his poetry collection, *The Rose that Grows from Concrete*, aware of the militant political activism of his family, including his mother Afeni Shakur and stepfather Mutulu. It was not until much later, however, that she learned of Mutulu Shakur's involvement in acupuncture.

Also in common with Parker-Rodgers, and with some of the students from POCA Tech, Garcia spent years as a social worker before settling on acupuncture as her approach to helping people in need. She spent time in Mexico, working at a nonprofit to help Central American immigrants and gaining a master's degree in human rights before moving to the Bronx. There she spent 10 years working with young people arrested for nonviolent offenses and victims of sex trafficking but eventually found herself carrying home too much emotional trauma and "totally burnt out." Garcia, who is Black, witnessed acupuncture as "really powerful" and "a great healing tool" in helping family members recover from ailments, but she still questioned its relevance to her community. It was her husband, an academic involved in the study of African diaspora and colonialism, who told her about Shakur's revolutionary acupuncture. She also met, on a trip to Cuba, Nehanda Abiodun, who was at BAAANA in the 1970s and had been living in exile since the fallout from the Brink's robbery of October 1981.

I grew up in San Francisco, California, in the 1980s. The geographical proximity to Oakland, California, the birthplace of the Black Panther Party, made revolutionary political movements for the liberation of Black and brown communities a palpable resource for me as young person. I didn't learn about [Black Panther cofounder] Bobby Seale, Angela Davis, or Mutulu Shakur in a classroom. Growing up Black in San Francisco, a city with the smallest African American population of any major city in the United States, taught me enough to pick up a book and fill in the gaps formal education left out. I remember hearing first-hand stories of political organizing by the adults in my life. These experiences informed me of basic truths I still hold to be true, that the oppression of Black and brown people not only in the United States, but globally, is a function of capitalism and white supremacy and must be dismantled by any means necessary. Every path I have taken in life, every career choice, including becoming an acupuncturist, has been informed by the history of revolutionary political movements centered in the liberation of Black and brown communities.

I first learned about Mutulu Shakur as a teenage fan of Tupac Shakur. Tupac's mother, Afeni Shakur, had been married to Mutulu Shakur, and the political influences of Tupac's upbringing in a militant family were also relayed in his poetry and music. But it wasn't until decades later that I would come across the name Mutulu Shakur as an acupuncturist. I learned about the occupation of Lincoln Hospital by the Young Lords and the opening of an acupuncture detox clinic after I had begun studying to become an acupuncturist. By this time I was living in the South Bronx, and had ended a decade-long career in the social work field, supporting Black and brown adults and youth overcome the barriers of trauma, incarceration, addiction, poverty, homelessness, sexual abuse, etcetera. Burnout from this tireless work led me to find a new route to heal self and the communities I have chosen to serve.

My husband was the first person who informed me about Black revolutionary movements that included acupuncture clinics, and this understanding was a major validation that the choice I had made to start a new career was relevant to the struggles of Black and brown people. I didn't learn anything of Mutulu Shakur's work as an acupuncturist in acupuncture school or in any formal setting; this [was] information I had to seek out independently. Being in school with the intention of becoming a doctor of acupuncture who provides high quality health care services to Black and brown communities at reduced cost or for free was a challenging choice. I was one of three Black students in my graduating cohort and the only student I knew who openly sought to return the knowledge of acupuncture to poor and working-class Black and brown communities.

In 2018, I had the opportunity to meet Nehanda Abiodun, a Black nationalist in political exile, in Havana, Cuba. In the 1970's Nehanda worked with Mutulu Shakur at the Lincoln Hospital Detox Clinic and later joined the Black Acupuncture Advisory Association of North America, Harlem's first acupuncture clinic. We spoke little about her acupuncture work, with the focus of conversation around the legacy of radical Black and brown liberation movements and how to apply those principles to the work we do today. My life's work, and by extension my career as an acupuncturist, is informed directly by Black militancy movements.[23]

Garcia added, "Of all the jobs I've had, I feel there's one united theme which is me showing up for people to try to support them to make the changes they want to manifest in their lives. Wanting to show up and ask what it is you want to work on, and to support that process. Wanting to discuss the way [to do that] so that you can manifest the changes each person is working for."[24]

Her words echo remarkably those voiced by members of POCA throughout my interviews and experience with them. They suggest a contemporary take on the same principles that drove the striking mental health workers under the Einstein/Lincoln Hospital affiliation (helping their client carry his bed out of the rat hole he was living in), the radical therapists (releasing people from rigid structural roles), the Lincoln Detox counselors, and the acupuncturists of Lincoln Detox, BAAANA, and First World Acupuncture. Each time the goal was to create social change by empowering people to free themselves from situations leading to physical and mental illness. Despite the significant social changes that have taken place since the 1970s, the challenge remains an unresolved imperative.

# Epilogue

The schism that occurred between the groups led by Michael Smith and Mutulu Shakur marked a turning point in the history of American acupuncture. Smith spent his life working within the system and prevailed, over the years becoming renowned as the chief developer and proponent of the acupuncture technique now known as the NADA protocol. Smith's achievement did not come easily. He was a tireless fighter who never shied from confrontation, and there was confrontation aplenty with Lincoln Hospital through the years. From his early action of exposing the medical chart of Carmen Rodriguez, the young woman who died of an abortion, to storming out of meetings with administrators decades later, Smith stood up for his beliefs and for the people who believed in him. Yet he was good at harnessing his own emotional energy; his storming was done in a calculated way.

Sonia Lopez, a medical doctor who began working at Lincoln in 1984, saw Smith's approach as highly effective. "As time wore on Mike got very involved with City Hall. Mike was a funny character," she said. "He was different but he knew how to sneak into very traditional people." Yet it was clear to Lopez that he could only have done so working from inside the system. "He had cultivated many friendships in City Hall—often he was treating people there or their families with acupuncture and they had benefited from it ... He was very smart and knew how to work with Lincoln and Health and Hospital Corporation to get things done. Mike knew how to work with people inside the system to keep a clinic open that was very much outside the system but inside Lincoln Hospital. I don't know how else it could have survived when the revolutionaries were no longer there."

While the people labeled "political" had left Lincoln, Lopez saw Smith's program as political. Using the Chinese medicine term referring to the relatively pacific side of things, she said, "His sense was you build the yin when the opposing forces are bigger than you. He was definitely—without using the political words—treating people as humans, treating a right-brain energy which was a political act. If you get enough people thinking that way, they won't be part of the system, or will be part of it differently."[1]

Smith engendered great loyalty in those who worked with him, some who began as community volunteers and had been with him for decades. Jeannette Robinson, who was a longtime administrator in Smith's department and is African American, said, "I saw him as a warrior. I saw him as Michael the archangel, but the warrior … He was our protector. And we were his." Carlos Alvarez, who as one of the first volunteers at Lincoln Detox had worked with Smith for 48 years, also viewed him as a defender: "Despite the threats of the hospital administration and others, Mike was a trooper. He had real big cojones—there is no doubt about that. I thought he was very fearless, really. He stayed the course, displaying real strengths. And he remained at Lincoln." Alvarez added, "He had no idea that he was this extraordinary human being, and he was an extraordinary human being who never acted that way. Mike forged a new path. He was on a mission to spread the work of NADA to the world."[2]

Some of Shakur's most ardent supporters view Smith in a different light, though. They see him as having come from the white-male, dominant medical paradigm to coopt a therapy Shakur and Bosque started. From their point of view, when they were evicted from the hospital, Smith did not support them. Instead, he took over acupuncture detox and willingly received credit for its development. "It's the age-old story that even a lot of acupuncture places, the first time you [visit] you had to go through a doctor first," said Haught. "It's all about power and control."[3] Bosque, who is more sanguine, said of Smith after the eviction, "I give him credit for keeping the program, but the politics was out of Lincoln, and we had to find other ways of doing what we do."[4]

Zeller takes a nuanced perspective. "He was very brilliant," she said of Smith. "But Mutulu and Walter [Bosque], they felt they had figured this whole thing out, they went to China and Montreal and studied acupuncture, they did it. So it was a real power struggle. The hospital, after the takeover, there were lots of community people on payroll. They did more political education, but they did total body acupuncture, which was not what was going on with Mike."[5]

There is little evidence that Smith gave credit to Shakur, Bosque, and the other revolutionary acupuncturists, aside from the article authored by him and Shakur in 1979. When asked, at a conference hosted by WCA, about the role of the Young Lords and Black Panthers in bringing acupuncture to Lincoln, he minimized its significance. At most, he credited them with opening up possibilities through the takeover of the hospital. "They gave us a certain freedom at the time of the 70s," he said.[6] But he characterized stories about the Young Lords as "mythology" and said, "most of the movement people were verbal people—acupuncture was all silent and mysterious so there was not a lot of simpatico, for the most part."[7]

The history of acupuncture detox is distorted by a false dichotomy. The dominant tale holds that only one group was truly interested in acupuncture (Smith's) while the other was only truly interested in revolution (Shakur's). But the truth is more complex: In fact, the revolutionaries were deeply in love with the idea and practice of acupuncture, while seeing acupuncture as a means to, and an expression of, revolution. Both fought the system in their ways—Smith as an MD within the hospital system (which had threatened to expel him), Shakur as an acupuncturist who was expelled by the system. Yet, for Shakur, his time working within the system was deeply meaningful. "Right now, today, you can go into New York City and in those municipal hospitals within black and Puerto Rican and poor communities—a municipal hospital, not a private hospital but the municipal hospital—you can now receive acupuncture treatment for drug withdrawal as an alternative method of treatment," he said. "I am proud to have been a part of the required effort and accomplishments making this possible. It means a lot to me and remains one of the most important periods of my life, guiding my human rights priorities. Those experiences completely reflect the narrative of my life's journey; both the good and the bad, absent the disinformation, misinformation and slander."[8]

Michael Smith died in December 2017; Mutulu Shakur remains in prison, where he has been for the last 35 years. In addition to the stroke he suffered in 2014, he has multiple chronic health problems, and like his mother he experiences vision problems due to glaucoma. On December 5, 2019, the Bureau of Prisons denied his legal team's request for compassionate release.

His situation was to worsen. In October 2019, Shakur was diagnosed with advanced bone cancer. He began receiving treatment while housed in the US Penitentiary in Victorville, California. A prisoner receiving medical treatment outside the prison loses even the shreds of dignity and autonomy afforded inside. According to Mark Kleiman, the lead attorney on the petition for compassionate release, Shakur was shackled to a bed while undergoing chemotherapy, surrounded by five security guards. In mid-winter, he was transferred without notice to a facility in Lexington, Kentucky. His legal team was denied access for 10 weeks. "We didn't know he was shackled to a bed. If someone is chained up in the forest, no one can hear him," said Kleiman.

In Lexington, Shakur was taken to an outside medical facility for chemotherapy, surrounded by five guards in the van on the way there and back as well as while getting infusions. Kleiman believes that, given the spike of coronavirus infections in Kentucky during that time, the close presence of the guards in confined spaces was "incredibly dangerous" for him. "The need for guards is purely imaginary and this aspect of his mistreatment is absolutely political," he said.[9] Indeed, Shakur contracted COVID-19 in early 2021 shortly after receiving a stem cell transplant, but he survived.

Judge Haight, the presiding judge who convicted Shakur, described his case as "an American tragedy."[10] It is a tragic irony that Shakur, who as a youthful revolutionary was dedicated to making the pursuit of health a human right, has been denied that right two generations on.

# Acknowledgements

I am indebted to many people who aided and abetted the writing of this book, none more than Anne Lown, who first sparked my interest and gave quiet encouragement along the way. Her casual mention of First World Acupuncture in a seemingly unrelated context sent me down a different path than I'd expected to be on, for which I'm most grateful.

My research was made infinitely more pleasant by the hospitality of Terue Tokoro, who provided a home base and a sympathetic ear during my trips to New York. Pat Benefiel went above and beyond her role as head librarian at the Pacific College of Health and Science in helping me acquire materials during the library's pandemic-enforced closure and sharing her memories of academia and leftist politics in the 1960s. Samantha Stevens of the Pacific College library was magically helpful in obtaining resources. Julie Chambers provided a critical link in connecting me with Mark Kleiman, who explained Mutulu Shakur's legal considerations; I am grateful to them both, and to Sean Gates of Yo San University Library for inviting me to speak at the meeting that led to that connection.

Heartfelt thanks to Franklin Apfel, Misha Cohen, Karen Cutler, Jackie Haught, Tatsuo Hirano, Sonia Lopez, Mario Wexu, and Barbara Zeller for sharing their experiences at Lincoln Detox, BAAANA, and First World Acupuncture, and to Lisa Rohleder, Skip Van Meter, and the students of POCA Tech for inviting me into their classroom to observe and talk about my research. The insight I gained from listening and speaking to "punks" at various POCA gatherings and at WCA was likewise invaluable. Tyler Phan was among the speakers at the Toronto POCAfest of 2018; I greatly appreciate his combination of academic rigor and enthusiastic iconoclasm, and for sharing his work as he turns his dissertation into a monograph. Ted Kaptchuk kindly took time from his monumental schedule to fill me in on the path that led him to Chinese medicine. I also want to thank the people who enriched my understanding of events in 1970s and 80s New York while speaking off the record.

Tenisha Dandridge, Monica Garcia, Felicia Parker-Rodgers, and Yvonne Scarlett generously gave of their time and inspired me with their personal histories and vision for the future. Margie Navarro was gracious in helping with communications to Mutulu Shakur. I am amazed and deeply grateful that Mutulu Shakur found the time to respond to my letters while in a clearly difficult situation in the US Penitentiary in Victorville.

Thanks to Elizabeth Demers of the University of Michigan Press for seeing the potential in this book and encouraging its development over the course of a year, and to the three anonymous reviewers whose thoughtful advice undoubtedly improved it. I'm most grateful to others who read individual chapters, including Claire McManus and Jess Gerber, and to Susan Reverby for finding time to read the final chapter's (more or less) final iteration and for sharing her insights into writing about revolutionary actions and actors.

Joanne Shwed (Backspace Ink) has been a meticulous grammarian and extraordinarily efficient designer and guiding light. My husband Matthew Binns is, among many other things, a skilled photo editor who saved the day more than once.

Finally, the thoughtful encouragement of my daughter Gabriela Navarro, and Matthew's unflagging support as he read, critiqued, asked questions, listened, and cooked meals, pulled me through as always.

# Notes

**PROLOGUE NOTE**

1. "Yes, Mr. Trump, Hurricane Maria Was a 'Real Catastrophe,'" *New York Times*, September 2, 2018, https://www.nytimes.com/2018/09/02/opinion/puerto-rico-hurricane-maria-death-toll.html.

**INTRODUCTION NOTES**

1. For instance, in Woody Allen's 1990 film, *Crimes and Misdemeanors*, in Jonathan Safran Foer's novel, *Here I Am* (New York: Farrar, Straus, and Giroux, 2016), and, indelibly, in Sam Lipsyte's 2019 novel, *Hark* (New York: Simon & Schuster, 2019).

2. Mei Zhan, *Other-Worldly: Making Chinese Medicine through Transnational Frames* (Durham: Duke University Press, 2009), 7-15.

3. Ibid., 31-34.

4. For example, the Black Acupuncturist Association established by acupuncturist/activist Tenisha Dandridge; see https://blackacupuncturist.org/.

5. A 2017 survey by the American Association of Acupuncture and Oriental Medicine, a national advocacy organization, found that 40 percent of respondents had assumed more than $100,000 in loans; see Amanda Gaitaud, "Stories of Struggle and Success: Looking at the Burden of Debt," *Acupuncture Today*, March 2018, vol. 19, issue 3.

6. For an analysis of American acupuncture education in the context of white supremacy culture, see Tyler Phan, "American Chinese Medicine" (PhD diss., University College London, 2017), https://discovery.ucl.ac.uk/id/eprint/1571107/.

7.  Johanna Fernández, *The Young Lords: A Radical History* (Chapel Hill: University of North Carolina Press, 2020), 5. Fernández describes how the 1960s generation of activists came to adopt revolutionary politics.

8.  The New Left rejected Old Left concepts, such as the centrality of class struggle, to emphasize other forms of oppression, like racism and sexism, and championed direct action and participatory democracy. Its broad range during a time of much social activism led to its being labeled a "movement of movements." See, for example, Van Gosse, *Rethinking the New Left: An Interpretive History* (New York: Palgrave Macmillan, 2005), esp. 1-8.

9.  Max Elbaum, *Revolution in the Air: Sixties Radicals Turn to Lenin, Mao, and Che* (New York: Verso, 2002, 2018), 2-3; Fernández, *The Young Lords*, 10.

10. Elbaum, *Revolution in the Air*, preface; Fernández, *The Young Lords*, 219. To the revolutionary healthcare activists, the lumpenproletariat signified heroin addicts, street people, and high school dropouts. See also Susan Reverby and Marsha Handelman, "Emancipation of Lincoln," *Health/PAC Bulletin*, Health Policy Advisory Center, no. 37, January 1972, 7.

11. The analysis was asserted in pamphlets such as Rodd Aya et al., *The Opium Trail: Heroin and Imperialism* (Somerville, MA: New England Free Press, April 1972) and Black Panther Michael Tabor's *Capitalism + Dope = Genocide*, which were popular among revolutionary activists. Michael Smith, a psychiatrist at Lincoln Hospital who was instrumental in developing and disseminating acupuncture for addiction, espoused a version of the analysis in "The Lily Connection: Drug Abuse and the Medical Profession" published in the magazine *Science for the People* (published by the radical scientists' movement of the same name) in 1978. Alfred W. McCoy exposed CIA involvement in trafficking in Southeast Asia in *The Politics of Heroin in Southeast Asia* (New York: Harper & Row, 1972) and in the same year was called to give testimony before the Foreign Operations Subcommittee of the Senate Appropriations Committee.

12. Fernández describes how the Young Lords purveyed the idea in the first edition of their newspaper as well as its intellectual origins and use as an educational tool in the radical drug detox program at Lincoln Hospital— see Fernández, *The Young Lords*, 220-221 and 303; Shakur frequently referred to it in strong terms, for example in Mutulu Shakur, "Dope is Death! Acupuncture Heals," BAAANA, June 29, 1976; in a speech given on March 18, 1979; and in Mutulu Shakur, "2018 Interview about Acupuncture & The Opioid Crisis," interview by Olga Khazan, Mutulu

Shakur, November 19, 2018, http://mutulushakur.com/site/2018/11/acupuncture-interview/.

13. Center for Substance Abuse Treatment (US), *Trauma-Informed Care in Behavioral Health Services*, Rockville (MD): Substance Abuse and Mental Health Services Administration (US), 2014 (Treatment Improvement Protocol (TIP) Series, no. 57). Appendix C, Historical Account of Trauma.

14. See Alondra Nelson, *Body and Soul: The Black Panther Party and the Fight Against Medical Discrimination* (Minneapolis: University of Minnesota Press, 2011), and Fernández, *The Young Lords*, esp. 135-154.

15. Fernández, *The Young Lords*, 3.

16. Elbaum, *Revolution in the Air*, preface.

17. Fernández, *The Young Lords*, 206. Fernández notes that 1960s radical activists used "the colonial experience" in a variety of ways to highlight and describe the experience of racial oppression within the United States.

18. Ibid., 201; Elbaum, *Revolution in the Air*, 48.

19. Julia Lovell, *Maoism: A Global History* (New York: Alfred A. Knopf, 2019), 125-126.

20. Mary Augusta Brazelton, *Mass Vaccination: Citizens' Bodies and State Power in Modern China* (Ithaca: Cornell University Press, 2019), 195-197. Brazelton contends that, seeking recognition as the sole leader of China, the People's Republic of China had to fend off competition from Taiwan's Republic of China in international circles. Providing aid to the nonaligned Third World nations was a way to curry favor when it came to recognition in bodies such as the United Nations and the WHO.

21. Jeremy Youde, "China's Health Diplomacy in Africa," *China: An International Journal*, 8, no. 1 (2010), 153.

22. Xiaoping Fang, *Barefoot Doctors and Western Medicine in China* (New York: University of Rochester Press, 2012), 47-51.

23. Brazelton, *Mass Vaccination*, 196; Alan Hutchison, *China's African Revolution* (Boulder, CO: Westview Press, 1975), 221-222.

24. Brazelton, *Mass Vaccination*, 198-199; Sung Lee, "WHO and the developing world: the contest for ideology," in *Western Medicine as Contested Knowledge*, eds.; Andrew Cunningham and Bridie Andrews (Manchester, UK: Manchester University Press, 1997), 24-43.

25. Brazelton, *Mass Vaccination*, 193; Hutchison, *China's African Revolution*, 221-222; Youde, "China's Health Diplomacy in Africa," 154.

26. Brazelton, *Mass Vaccination*, 187.

27. Declaration of Alma-Ata, International Conference on Primary Health Care, Alma-Ata, USSR, 6-12, September 1978.

28. Ibid., 193, 198. Brazelton argues that revolutionary China has been underrecognized for its role in getting primary care as a health strategy accepted on the world stage, in part because it did not send a delegation to Alma-Ata—held on Soviet territory, at the USSR's insistence—due to the continuing Sino-Soviet schism. For a comprehensive analysis of China's rural healthcare model on the declaration of Alma-Ata, see Sung Lee, "WHO and the developing world: the contest for ideology."

29. From a search of Newspapers.com, May 14, 2019.

30. Kim Taylor, "The History of the Barefoot Doctors" (unpublished MPhil. thesis, University of Cambridge, 1994), 22.

31. Robert S. Elegant (*Los Angeles Times*), "'Barefoot Doctors' Replace Practitoners [sic] in Red China," *Lansing State Journal*, November 28, 1968. The claims were far from the truth. In fact, urban areas of China continued to rely on a hospital-based, Western style of medicine, while in rural areas a three-tiered system prevailed, consisting of brigade medical stations, commune clinics, and barefoot doctors. A key role of barefoot doctors and the commune clinics was to give outside referrals to medical doctors where necessary. See Fang, *Barefoot Doctors*, 132-150.

32. Julian Schuman, "The Barefoot Doctors: China's Crash-Course Physicians Tend the Peasants," *Palm Beach Post-Times*, July 25, 1971. Notably, this article was published the day before journalist James Reston's famous article, describing his experience with postappendectomy acupuncture while accompanying Henry Kissinger in China, appeared in the *New York Times*. Reston's article is frequently attributed with having ignited American interest in acupuncture.

33. Julia Lovell contends that Nixon's visit itself was a consequence of the Sino-Soviet split. See Lovell, *Maoism*, 126.

34. "China's 'Barefoot Doctors' Produce Medical Revolution," *Asbury Park Press*, May 24, 1973.

35. "China's 'Barefoot Doctors' Win Praise from 2 U.S. Physicians," *The Greenville News*, July 9, 1973.

36. Victor W. Sidel, "Barefoot Doctors of the People's Republic of China," *New England Journal of Medicine*, 286, no. 24, 1972, 1293. Sidel was accompanied by his wife Ruth, a psychiatric social worker. Together the Sidels wrote several publications based on their impressions, including the book *Serve the People: Observations on Medicine in the People's Republic of China* (New York: Josiah Macy, Jr. Foundation, 1973). Brazelton (*Mass*

*Vaccination*, 204) notes that the Sidels had Communist leanings before their visit. Sidel was also affiliated with the Department of Community Health at Albert Einstein College of Medicine, Lincoln Hospital's paternal affiliate under the Affiliation Program. Montefiore would develop its own acupuncture program for community care in the 1980s.

37. Paul G. Pickowicz, "Barefoot Doctors in China: People, Politics, and Paramedicine," in *Modern China and Traditional Chinese Medicine*, ed. Guenter B. Risse (Springfield, IL: Charles C. Thomas, Publisher, 1973), 126. White wrote a short piece for the *New York Times* of his impressions of China's healthcare system: "China's Heart is in the Right Place," *New York Times*, December 5, 1971.

38. Pickowicz, "Barefoot Doctors in China," 126; Guenter B. Risse, "Introduction," in *Modern China and Traditional Chinese Medicine*, ed. Risse, 100.

39. Fang, *Barefoot Doctors*, 99, 101-105. A central thesis of Fang's book is that the barefoot doctors facilitated the spread of biomedicine throughout China by introducing Western pharmaceuticals such as antibiotics to rural residents, who came to prefer them to the slower-acting Chinese herbs.

40. Ibid., 47; Pickowicz, "Barefoot Doctors in China," 133.

41. Fang, *Barefoot Doctors,* 49-54; Pickowicz, "Barefoot Doctors in China," 134.

42. Fang, *Barefoot Doctors*, 51-54.

43. Tatsuo Hirano, telephone interview with the author, August 15, 2020.

44. Fang, *Barefoot Doctors*, 152-153; Sidel, "Barefoot Doctors of the People's Republic of China," 1293; Taylor, "The History of the Barefoot Doctors," 18. Fang states that the barefoot doctors were deliberately chosen from the peasant class, categorized for statistical purposes as peasants, and required to continue work in agriculture.

45. Anne Lown, telephone interview with the author, September 26, 2017.

46. Franklin Apfel, telephone interview with the author, May 27, 2019; David Werner, David and Carol Thurman, and Jane Maxwell, *Where There Is No Doctor: A Village Health Care Handbook* (Berkeley, CA: Hesperian Health Guides, 1977). The book was first published in Spanish as *Donde No Hay Doctor* in 1970.

47. *A Barefoot Doctor's Manual: The American Translation of the Official Chinese Paramedical Manual* (Philadelphia, PA: Running Press, 1977). Brazelton (*Mass Vaccination*, 198-199) notes that the manual was first published in English by the John E. Fogarty International Center for

Advanced Study in the Health Sciences, a division of the NIH dedicated to global health.

48. "The RW Interview: 'Dr. Tolbert Small: Journey of a People's Doctor,'" *Revolutionary Worker* #1139, February 17, 2002, https://revcom.us/a/ v23/1130-39/1139/drsmall.htm; news briefs, *Los Angeles Times*, March 10, 1972, 2.

49. "Black Panther Members on Way to China," *Los Angeles Times*, March 6, 1972; Angela Davis, *Angela Davis: An Autobiography* (New York: International Publishers, 1988), 302.

50. "The RW Interview: 'Dr. Tolbert Small.'"

51. Sean Hsiang-Lin Lei, *Neither Donkey nor Horse: Medicine in the Struggle Over China's Modernity* (London: University of Chicago Press, 2014), 228-238, esp. 231; Fang, *Barefoot Doctors*, 163; Liping Bu, "From Public Health to State Medicine: John B. Grant and China's Health Profession," *Harvard Asia Quarterly*, 13, no. 4 (2012), 8-15.

52. Bu, "From Public Health to State Medicine," 26-34. John B. Grant, who was born and raised in China but received his medical training at the University of Michigan and his public health degree from Johns Hopkins University, was appointed Professor and Head of the Department of Hygiene and Public Health at PUMC in 1924. (The Rockefeller Foundation modeled PUMC on the medical college of Johns Hopkins.) Bu argues that Grant's ideas, including that healthcare was "most efficiently achieved through an integration of preventive and curative medicine in a community health service," have had a lasting influence on China across political systems.

53. Lei, *Neither Donkey nor Horse*, 232-233.

54. Ibid., 231-238.

55. Bridie Andrews, *The Making of Modern Chinese Medicine, 1850-1960* (Honolulu: University of Hawaii Press, 2014), 110.

56. Lei, *Neither Donkey nor Horse*, 231-232.

57. Risse makes a similar point in *Modern China and Traditional Chinese Medicine*, stating, "Our rural areas and inner city ghettoes could greatly benefit from a decentralized system of medical care delivered in part by paramedical people recruited from these areas," 100.

58. Apfel, interview; Fitzhugh Mullan, *White Coat, Clenched Fist: The Political Education of an American Physician* (Ann Arbor: University of Michigan Press, 1976, 2006), 98-99.

59. Fang, *Barefoot Doctors*, 160, referencing Reinhard Spree, *Health and Social Class in Imperial Germany: A Social History of Mortality, Morbidity and Inequality* (New York: St. Martin's Place, 1988), 158; Paul Root Wolpe, "The Maintenance of Professional Authority: Acupuncture and the American Physician," *Social Problems*, 32, no. 5 (1985), 409-424, https://doi.org/10.2307/800772. Wolpe discusses the terms cultural authority and social authority as two forms of control through which professions maintain their dominance. Cultural authority involves construction of realities and their concomitant values and meanings, while social authority encompasses actual legislation to embed cultural constructs into institutions.

60. Fang, *Barefoot Doctors*, 160-176, esp. 160-161.

61. For more insight into the regulation and suppression of acupuncture in the American healthcare system, see Wolpe, "The Maintenance of Professional Authority: Acupuncture and the American Physician," and Linda Barnes, "The Acupuncture Wars: The Professionalizing of American Acupuncture—A View from Massachusetts," *Medical Anthropology*, 22, no. 3, 261-301.

62. Theodore Roszak, *The Making of a Counter Culture: Reflections on the Technocratic Society and its Youthful Opposition* (Garden City, NY: Anchor Books, 1969), 35.

63. Miguel "Mickey" Melendez, *We Took the Streets: Fighting for Latino Rights with the Young Lords* (New York: St. Martin's Press, 2003), 86-87; Nelson, *Body and Soul*, 82-84.

64. The free clinic movement, which began with the Haight-Ashbury Free Medical Clinic in 1967, initially served mainly hippies and other disaffected white youth. However, there was a push to make it relevant to people of color, particularly Black Americans, as well. See Gregory Swart, "The Free Clinic Movement," in *The Free Clinic: A Community Approach to Health Care and Drug Abuse*, eds. David E. Smith, David J. Bentel, and Jerome L. Schwartz (Beloit, WI: Stash Press, 1971), 92-98, and Harry W. Clark, "How Relevant is the Free Clinic Movement to Black People," *Journal of Social Issues*, 30, no. 1, 1974, 67-72.

65. Tamara Venit Shelton, *Herbs and Roots: A History of Chinese Doctors in the American Medical Marketplace* (New Haven: Yale University Press, 2019), 233-234.

66. Misha Cohen, telephone interview with the author, December 8, 2019; Mao and his acolytes also promulgated a close relationship between dialectical materialism and Chinese medicine: see "Mao Tse-Tung, 1967, 1:314," quoted in Paul U. Unschuld, *Medicine in China: A History of Ideas*

(Berkeley: University of California Press, 1985), 254, and Jen K'ang T'ung, "Dialectic in Acupuncture Anesthesia," 1974, 63-64, quoted in Unschuld, *Medicine in China*, 255.

67. Venit Shelton, *Herbs and Roots*, 202.

68. For a description of the complex relationship between traditional Chinese herbalists and biomedicine, see Venit Shelton, *Herbs and Roots*, 200-218. At least one American-born herbalist described chiropractic as an option not only for its licensure but because it combined Western-style diagnosis with an understanding of holism and energy flow—an ideal combination of traditional Chinese medicine and biomedicine.

69. Ibid., 217.

70. James Reston, "Now About My Operation in Peking," *New York Times*, July 26, 1971, https://www.nytimes.com/1971/07/26/archives/now-about-my-operation-in-peking-now-let-me-tell-you-about-my.html.

71. Jane Brody, "Acupuncture Demonstrated at Medical Parley Here," *New York Times*, December 15, 1971, https://www.nytimes.com/1971/12/15/archives/acupuncture-demonstrated-at-medical-parley-here.html. Brody's conclusion was in line with the scientific community and was likely a reflection of the milieu from which she was reporting.

72. This spectacular swing in perception preceded what Mei Zhan describes as a translocal wave beginning in the 1980s. The wave shifted the focus on traditional Chinese medicine practices from poor rural populations in developing countries to relatively prosperous populations in the developed world. In the process, preventive medicine was redefined, from basic primary care to general mind-body wellness. See Zhan, *Other-Worldly*, 14-15.

73. C. Robert Jennings, "The Needle Epidemic," *Los Angeles Times*, October 1, 1972.

74. Brazelton, *Mass Vaccination*, 186.

75. Wolpe, "The Maintenance of Professional Authority: Acupuncture and the American Physician," 411.

76. Barbara J. Culliton, "Acupuncture: Fertile Ground for Faddists and Serious NIH Research," *Science*, 177, no. 4049 (1972), 592.

77. Nobuko Miyamoto tells her own story as a Japanese American activist and artist in *Not Yo' Butterfly: My Long Song of Relocation, Race, Love, and Revolution* (Oakland: University of California Press, 2021).

78. Hirano, interview.

## CHAPTER 1 NOTES

1. Miguel "Mickey" Melendez, *We Took the Streets: Fighting for Latino Rights with the Young Lords* (New York: St. Martin's Press, 2003), 35-36.

2. Mel Rosenthal, *In the South Bronx of America* (Willimantic, CT: Curbstone Press, 2000), 32-33.

3. Walter Bosque was speaking on a panel at the Colegio de Abogados in San Juan, Puerto Rico, headed "Salud, Dignidad, y Pobreza: Un Asunto de Derechos Humanos" ("Health, Dignity, and Poverty: A Matter of Human Rights"). Attended by the author on April 18, 2018.

4. Rosenthal, *In the South Bronx of America*, 18.

5. Deborah Wallace and Rodrick Wallace, *A Plague on Your Houses: How New York Was Burned Down and National Public Health Crumbled* (New York: Verso, 1998), 21-22. The Moynihan quote is from "Text of the Moynihan Memorandum on the Status of Negroes," *New York Times*, January 1970. Moynihan's text also linked "fires in the black slums" to "the urban riots of 1964-1968," suggesting another purpose for the policy of benign neglect.

6. Wallace and Wallace, *A Plague on Your Houses*, 25-26. The two main fallacies the Wallaces cite regarding planned shrinkage were: 1) the policy had already been in use for some time before it became official and was indeed the cause behind some of the targeted areas' failure; and 2) it was based on an unproven theory that cities have a natural life cycle ending in death.

7. Ibid., xvi.

8. Marshall Berman, "Emerging from the Ruins," *Dissent Magazine*, Winter 2014, https://www.dissentmagazine.org/article/emerging-from-the-ruins.

9. Marshall Berman, *All That Is Solid Melts into Air: The Experience of Modernity* (New York: Penguin Books, 1988), 307.

10. Robert A. Caro, *The Power Broker: Robert Moses and the Fall of New York* (New York: Vintage Books, 1975), 878.

11. Ibid., 850-884, esp. 877-878.

12. Berman, *All That Is Solid Melts into Air*, 293.

13. Wallace and Wallace, *A Plague on Your Houses*, 11-14.

14. Frances Perkins, "Oral History Reminiscences" (Columbia University Collection), quoted in Berman, *All That is Solid Melts into Air*, 304. Perkins, Franklin Delano Roosevelt's Secretary of Labor, who worked closely with Moses and was said to admire him, was disturbed to find

his attitude to people themselves. "To him they were lousy, dirty people, throwing bottles all over Jones Beach. 'I'll get them! I'll teach them!'"

15. Wallace and Wallace, *A Plague on Your Houses*, 16. The authors do not cite any specific evidence to support this rather spectacular claim but connect it implicitly to the weakening of community structures amid the experience of loss and displacement caused by Moses' projects.

16. Ibid., 17.

17. Berman, *All That Is Solid Melts into Air*, 325.

18. *Man Alive*, season 7, episode 1, "The Bronx is Burning," BBC Television and Time-Life Films, aired September 27, 1972.

19. Rosenthal, *In the South Bronx of America*, 17, 37, 70.

20. *The Police Tapes*, directed by Alan and Susan Raymond. Video Vérité, 1977, https://www.youtube.com/watch?v=xfE4NjiJtiA.

21. *The Fire Next Door*, directed by Tom Spain. *CBS Reports with Bill Moyers*, 1977, https://www.youtube.com/watch?v=RQkhD-2cWwY; Rosenthal, *In the South Bronx of America*, 51.

22. *The Fire Next Door*.

23. Bouza was also a critic of the investigation of Malcolm X's assassination. Decades later, he wrote, "The investigation was botched." Quoted by John Leland, "Pressure Builds to Reinvestigate the 1965 Killing of Malcolm X," *New York Times*, February 9, 2020, https://www.nytimes.com/2020/02/06/nyregion/malcolm-x-assassination-case-reopened.html. See also *Who Killed Malcolm X*, directed by Rachel Dretzin and Phil Bertelsen. Fusion, 2020. Streamed on Netflix.

24. *The Police Tapes*. This was the era of Michael Armstrong's crackdown on police corruption as chief counsel to the Knapp Commission, appointed in response to the whistleblowing of two officers, David Durk and Frank Serpico. The commission uncovered systemic corruption among New York City police. Armstrong quoted Serpico as saying, "Ten percent of the department is absolutely corrupt, 10 percent is absolutely honest and the other 80 percent, they wish they were honest." Quoted by Sam Roberts, "Michael Armstrong Dies at 86; Fought Police Corruption in New York," *New York Times*, October 22, 2019, https://www.nytimes.com/2019/10/21/nyregion/michael-armstrong-dead.html.

25. *Lincoln Hospital: A Film by Newsreel*, Third World Newsreel, 1970.

26. Robb Burlage, "Bronxmanship," *Health/PAC Bulletin*, Health Policy Advisory Center, April 1969, 4.

27. The following synopsis of Lincoln Hospital's history is based on Fitzhugh Mullan's account in *White Coat, Clenched Fist: The Political Education of an American Physician* (Ann Arbor: University of Michigan Press, 1976, 2006), 117-121.

28. Ibid., 121-122.

29. Susan Reverby and Marsha Handelman, "Emancipation of Lincoln," *Health/PAC Bulletin*, no. 37, January 1972, 13.

30. Mullan, *White Coat, Clenched Fist*, 125-126; Melendez, *We Took the Streets*, 162-168. Both Mullan and Melendez feature chapters titled "The Butcher Shop."

31. Reverby and Handelman, "Emancipation of Lincoln," 2-3.

32. Mullan, *White Coat, Clenched Fist*, 110-113.

33. Reverby and Handelman, "Emancipation of Lincoln," 2-3.

34. Barbara and John Ehrenreich, eds., *The American Health Empire: Power, Profits and Politics. A Report from the Health Policy Advisory Center (Health/PAC)* (New York: Vintage Books, 1970), 14.

35. Ibid., 40-49; for a deconstruction of the Einstein-Montefiore medical empire, see "The Trouble with Empires," *Health/PAC Bulletin*, Health Policy Advisory Center, April 1969.

36. Barbara Ehrenreich, "Giving Power to the People: The Early Days of Health/PAC," *Health/PAC Bulletin,* Health Policy Advisory Center, 18, no. 4, Winter 1988, 5.

37. Barbara Ehrenreich, "Bronx Community Wants Control," *Health/PAC Bulletin*, Health Policy Advisory Center, September 1970, 13.

38. Robb Burlage, *New York City's Municipal Hospitals: A Policy Review* (Washington, DC: Institute for Policy Studies, 1967).

39. Burlage, "Bronxmanship," 5; Ehrenreich, eds., *The American Health Empire*, 85.

40. Ehrenreich, eds., *The American Health Empire*, 63.

41. *Lincoln Hospital: A Film by Newsreel.*

42. Maxine Kenny, "Taking Care of their Own," *Health/PAC Bulletin*, Health Policy Advisory Center, April 1969, 13; Ehrenreich, eds., *The American Health Empire*, 255-256.

43. Franklin Apfel, telephone interview with the author, May 27, 2019.

44. Sonia Lopez, telephone interview with the author, March 25, 2019.

45. Kenny, "Taking Care of their Own," 13.

46. "'Barefoot Doctors' Replace Practitoners [sic] in Red China," *Lansing State Journal*, November 28, 1968.

47. Jackie Haught, telephone interview with the author, May 5, 2019, and Tatsuo Hirano, telephone interview with the author, August 15, 2020. Haught and Hirano both categorically defined "love for the people" as a primary motivation in the movement. They particularly ascribed this motivation to Mutulu Shakur. Their words were supported by statements other revolutionary acupuncturists made to me about the purpose of their practice. "Love for the people" was also a phrase used by Shakur in reference to Black militancy.

48. "The Encyclopedia of Anti-Revisionism On-Line," transcription, editing and markup by Paul Saba, first published in *The Guardian*, December 27, 1972. https://www.marxists.org/history/erol/ncm-1/hrum.htm; Reverby and Handelman, "Emancipation of Lincoln," 4; Mullan, *White Coat, Clenched Fist,* 193-195.

49. "Editorial: Institutional Organizing," *Health/PAC Bulletin*, Health Policy Advisory Center, no. 37, January 1972, 1-7; Mullan, *White Coat, Clenched Fist*, 185-186.

50. Ehrenreich, "Bronx Community Wants Control," 13; Reverby and Handelman, "Emancipation of Lincoln," 7.

51. Ehrenreich, "Bronx Wants Community Control," 13-14.

52. Melendez, *We Took the Streets*, 167.

53. Mullan, *White Coat, Clenched Fist*, 152. Mullan describes the recruitment brochure for the collective; its stated aim was to accrue a "critical mass" of socially conscious medics to enact meaningful change at Lincoln Hospital.

54. Alondra Nelson, *Body and Soul: The Black Panther Party and the Fight Against Medical Discrimination* (Minneapolis: University of Minnesota Press, 2011), 87; Mullan, *White Coat, Clenched Fist*, 195.

55. Mullan, *White Coat, Clenched Fist*, 164.

56. Melendez, *We Took the Streets*, 170.

57. Daniel O'Grady, "Radicals End Hospital Seizure as Cops Mass," *Daily News*, July 15, 1970.

58. Mutulu Shakur, "2018 Interview about Acupuncture & The Opioid Crisis," interview by Olga Khazan, on mutulushakur.com, posted November 19, 2018, http://mutulushakur.com/site/2018/11/acupuncture-interview/.

59. Mullan, *White Coat, Clenched Fist*, 147; Ehrenreich, "Bronx Community Wants Control," 14.

60. Mullan, *White Coat, Clenched Fist*, 150; Harry Schwartz, "Hospital Target for a Test by Radicals," *New York Times*, September 6, 1970, https://www.nytimes.com/1970/09/06/archives/hospital-target-for-a-test-by-radicals.html.

61. Michael T. Kaufman, "Lincoln Hospital: Case History of Dissension that Split Staff," *New York Times*, December 21, 1970, https://www.nytimes.com/1970/12/21/archives/lincoln-hospital-case-history-of-dissension-that-split-staff.html.

62. Ibid.; Mullan, *White Coat, Clenched Fist*, 165-166.

63. Kaufman, "Lincoln Hospital: Case History of Dissention that Split Staff."

64. Schwartz, "Hospital Target for a Test by Radicals."

65. Franklin Apfel, email communication with the author, May 2, 2019.

66. "Lincoln O.D.'s on T.P.F.," *Health/PAC Bulletin*, Health Policy Advisory Center, December 1970; Mullan, *White Coat, Clenched Fist*, 150-151.

67. Ellinor R. Mitchell, *Fighting Drug Abuse with Acupuncture: The Treatment that Works* (Berkeley, CA: Pacific View Press, 1995), 37-38. Mitchell writes that a matching grant of $1,128,388 was provided by the New York State Narcotics Addiction Control Commission; the city could match it with cash or in-kind goods and services. The program operated largely on volunteer work until the full funding arrived six months later.

68. Alfred W. McCoy, with Catherine B. Read and Leonard P. Adams II, *The Politics of Heroin in Southeast Asia* (New York: Harper & Row, 1972), 7.

69. Ibid., 8.

70. Ibid., 14.

71. Testimony by Alfred W. McCoy on the Heroin Traffic in Southeast Asia before the Foreign Operations Subcommittee of the Senate Appropriations Committee on 2 June 1972, https://www.cia.gov/library/readingroom/docs/CIA-RDP74B00415R000400020015-6.pdf.

72. Johanna Fernández, *The Young Lords: A Radical History* (Chapel Hill: University of North Carolina Press, 2020), 220-221. Fernández also argues that the Young Lords' efforts to combat drug addiction were ultimately harmful to the organization for two principal reasons: Rehabilitation was too resource-intensive and diverted energy from grassroots political organizing to social services; and the embracing of unreliable members of the lumpenproletariat (including the drug users being rehabilitated) made the organization vulnerable to infiltration by the FBI, who were known to use lumpens as agents provocateurs.

73. *The Black Power Mixtape 1967-1975*. Directed by Goran Hugo Olsson, release date February 2011.

74. Wallace and Wallace, *A Plague on Your Houses*, 113-114, 120-121.

75. Barbara Zeller, telephone interview with the author, April 19, 2019.

76. Fernández, *The Young Lords*, 220. Fernández writes that the Bronx had the world's highest rate of heroin addiction.

77. James Reston, "Now About My Operation in Peking," *New York Times*, July 26, 1971, https://www.nytimes.com/1971/07/26/archives/now-about-my-operation-in-peking-now-let-me-tell-you-about-my.html.

78. Michael Smith, "The Lilly Connection: Drug Abuse and the Medical Profession," in *Science for the People*, 10, no. 1, January/February 1978, 11.

79. Ibid., 12; Rodd Aya et al., *The Opium Trail: Heroin and Imperialism* (Somerville, MA: New England Free Press, April 1972), 72.

80. Murray Kempton, *The Briar Patch: The People of the State of New York v. Lumumba Shakur et al.* (New York: E. P. Dutton Co., Inc., 1973), 126. Kempton describes Tabor, a member of the Panther 21 who had just been released on bail, talking to addicts who were occupying Harlem Hospital to demand detoxification services. He quotes Tabor: "And you'll do this too if you have to; you will have just traded habits and now you are a slave to the state."

81. Misha Cohen, telephone interview with the author, December 8, 2019.

82. Peter Bourne, Department of Justice and the Law Enforcement Assistance Administration, *The Methadone Maintenance Treatment Manual*, 5, as quoted in Smith, "The Lilly Connection," 13, and in Mutulu Shakur, "Dope is Death: Acupuncture Heals!," The Black Acupuncture Advisory Association of North America, Inc., New York, June 1976, 3.

83. Smith, "The Lilly Connection," 9.

84. Shakur, "2018 Interview about Acupuncture & the Opioid Crisis."

85. McCoy, *The Politics of Heroin in Southeast Asia*, 2.

86. Ibid., 3-4.

87. Ibid., referencing United Nations Department of Social Affairs, *Bulletin on Narcotics*, 3-4, 6, 7, 26.

88. Aya et al., *The Opium Trail*.

89. Ibid., 47-64.

90. Melendez, *We Took the Streets*, 177.

91. Aya et al., *The Opium Trail*.

92. Horn's work was also popular with radical doctors, medical students, and others involved in healthcare and leftist politics. In addition to his book, Horn gave lecture tours in the United States. See Susan M. Reverby, *Co-Conspirator for Justice: The Revolutionary Life of Dr. Alan Berkman* (Chapel Hill: University of North Carolina Press, 2020), 76.

93. Melendez, *We Took the Streets*, 177.


## CHAPTER 2 NOTES

1. Initially, the language signed by California Governor Jerry Brown in two measures, SB951 and AB1453, on September 30, 2012, stated that patients would be charged a $30 copayment for acupuncture services for "nausea and chronic pain." However, in practice copayments and covered conditions vary wildly across plans. In my own practice, copayments have ranged from nil to $60 (more than the practitioner's reimbursement), some patients are allowed unlimited annual treatments, some have an annual or monthly cap, and others have a theoretical allowance contingent on submission of periodical "medical necessity" reviews. Regarding conditions, different plans allow coverage of various International Disease Classification codes. Some offer a broad range while others are more restrictive; in the case of one plan, acupuncture covered one circumstance only—in lieu of anesthesia during surgery—a rather bizarre anachronism in the twenty-first century.

2. C. M. Cassidy, "Chinese Medicine Users in the United States. Part I: Utilization, Satisfaction, Medical Plurality," *Journal of Alternative and Complementary Medicine*, 4, no. 1 (1996): 17-27; Kimberley M. Tippens et al., "Patient Perspectives on Care Received at Community Acupuncture Clinics: A Qualitative Thematic Analysis," *BMC Complementary and Alternative Medicine*, 13, no. 293 (2013), http://www.biomedcentral.com/1472-6882/13/293.

3. Centers for Medicare and Medicaid Services, "Decision Memo for Acupuncture for Chronic Low Back Pain (CAG-00452N)," https://www.cms.gov/medicare-coverage-database/details/nca-decision-memo.aspx?NCAId=295.

4. Arthur Yin Fan et al., "Distribution of Licensed Acupuncturists and Educational Institutions in the United States at the Start of 2018," *Complementary Therapies in Medicine*, 41 (2018): 295-301.

5. Ibid., 295.

6. Ibid.

7. "Decision Memo for Acupuncture for Chronic Low Back Pain (CAG-00452N)," Centers for Medicare & Medicaid Services, https://www.cms.gov/medicare-coverage-database/details/nca-decision-memo.aspx?NCAId=295.

8. Sam Collins speaking at the NCCAOM-ASA Weekly Town Hall, June 24, 2020, https://www.nccaom.org/nccaom-webinars-posted/townhalls-meetings/. Two professional organizations, the NCCAOM and the Oriental Medicine and the American Society of Acupuncturists, held weekly online town hall meetings during the first months of the coronavirus pandemic to brief acupuncturists on new information. Collins is director of the American Acupuncture Council Insurance Information Networks.

9. A medical acupuncture course, required in a few states and the District of Columbia for a physician to practice acupuncture, mandates 200-300 hours of training. The majority of states allow MDs to perform acupuncture within their scope of practice, while three states (Hawaii, Montana, and New Mexico) require that MDs obtain a license through the same path as licensed acupuncturists. See Katerina Lin and Cynthia Tung, "The Regulation of the Practice of Acupuncture by Physicians in the United States," *Medical Acupuncture*, 3, no. 29 (2017). NCCAOM, "Educational Requirements for NCCAOM Certification," https://www.nccaom.org/certification/nccaom-certification-eligibility/educational-eligibility/ and Department of Consumer Affairs Acupuncture Board Exam Requirements.

10. Acupuncture.Com—Gateway to Chinese Medicine, Health and Wellness/State Laws, http://www.acupuncture.com/statelaws/stelaws.htm.

11. Neiguan, or Pericardium 6 (P6), is one of the most-researched acupuncture points because of its documented effects on nausea and hot flashes—two conditions that affect women being treated for breast cancer or menopausal symptoms, which are themselves intensively researched. In Chinese medicine, P6 is also a primary point for treating chest pain or heart conditions. For research on its antiemetic effects, see for example Guo-Shiou Liao, Maria Karmella Apaya, and Lie-Fen Shyur, "Herbal Medicine and Acupuncture for Breast Cancer Palliative Care and Adjuvant Therapy," *Evidence-Based Complementary and Alternative Medicine* (2013), http://dx.doi.org/10.1155/2013/437948; Siwoo Lee et al., "Electroacupuncture on P6 Prevents Opioid-Induced Nausea and Vomiting after Laparoscopic Surgery," *Chinese Journal of Integrative Medicine*, 19, 4 (2013), doi: 10.1007/s11655-013-1425-7; A. Molassiotis et al., "The Effects of P6 Acupressure in the Prophylaxis of Chemotherapy-Related Nausea and Vomiting in Breast Cancer Patients," *Complementary Therapies in Medicine*, 15, 1 (2006), doi:10.1016/j.ctim.2006.07.005; and

Andrew Vickers, "Can Acupuncture Antiemesis Have Specific Effects on Health? A Systematic Review of Acupuncture Antiemesis Trials," in *Journal of the Royal Society of Medicine*, 89, no. 6 (1996): 303-311.

12. For example, the "balancing" systems of Master Tung and Richard Tan; the Korean hand system; Japanese hara diagnosis; and several different interpretations of ear needling.

13. For a full analysis of "scientizing Chinese medicine" under the Nationalist government, see Sean Hsiang-Lin Lei, *Neither Donkey nor Horse: Medicine in the Struggle Over China's Modernity* (London: University of Chicago Press, 2014), chapter 7, 141-166.

14. Ibid., 148. Lei describes this as an implication of the project.

15. Tyler Phan, "American Chinese Medicine" (PhD diss., University College London, 2017), https://discovery.ucl.ac.uk/id/eprint/1571107/, 79-85.

16. Department of Consumers Affairs, Acupuncture Board, "Acupuncture Board History," https://www.acupuncture.ca.gov/about_us/history.shtml.

17. Steven Rosenblatt and Keith Kirts, *The Birth of Acupuncture in America: The White Crane's Gift* (Bloomington, IN: Balboa Press, 2016), 146, as quoted in Phan, "American Chinese Medicine," 107.

18. C. Norman Shealy, "A Physiological Basis for Electro-Acupuncture," in *Modern China and Traditional Chinese Medicine*, ed. Guenter B. Risse (Springfield, IL: Charles C. Thomas, Publisher, 1973), 89.

19. Elisabeth Hsu, "Innovations in Acumoxa: Acupuncture Analgesia, Scalp and Ear Acupuncture in the People's Republic of China," *Social Science and Medicine*, 42, no. 3 (1996), 421-430, esp. 422-424.

20. Paul Pickowicz, *A Sensational Encounter with High Socialist China* (Hong Kong: City University of Hong Kong, 2019), 92. Photos on 53 and 99.

21. Ibid., 101.

22. "Mao Tse-Tung, 1967, 1:314," quoted in Paul U. Unschuld, *Medicine in China: A History of Ideas* (Berkeley: University of California Press, 1985), 254.

23. Unschuld, *Medicine in China*, 255.

24. Keng Hsi-Chen and T'ao Nai-huang, "The Evaluation of Acupuncture Anesthesia Must Seek Truth from Facts," in Unschuld, *Medicine in China*, 360-366.

25. Ibid.

26. Hsu, "Innovations in Acumoxa," 424.

27. Lei, *Neither Donkey nor Horse*, 158.

28. Gwei-Djen Lu and Joseph Needham, *Celestial Lancets* (Cambridge: Cambridge University Press, 1980), quoted in Hsu, "Innovations in Acumoxa," 423.

29. Lei, *Neither Donkey nor Horse*, 159.

30. Bridie Andrews, *The Making of Modern Chinese Medicine, 1850-1960* (Honolulu: University of Hawaii Press, 2014), 203.

31. Ibid., 201-203.

32. Weidong Lu, "Developing Oncology Acupuncture, a New Subspecialty, at a Harvard Cancer Hospital," Acupuncture Research Resource Center, last modified April 2, 2019, https://www.acupunctureresearch.org.uk/symposium/symposium-archive/item/374-developing-oncology-acupuncture-a-new-subspecialty-at-a-harvard-cancer-hospital-weidong-lu.html.

33. Han's studies and reviews in this area are too numerous to list; they include, for example, J. S. Han and G. X. Xie, "Dynorphin: Important Mediator for Electroacupuncture Analgesia in the Spinal Cord of the Rabbit," *Pain*, 18 (1984): 367-377; J. S. Han, "Differential Release of Enkephalin and Dynorphin by Low and High Frequency Electroacupuncture in the Central Nervous System," *Acupuncture Science International Journal*, 1 (1990): 19-27; and J. S. Han, "Opioid and Anti-Opioid Peptides: A Model of Yin-Yang Balance in Acupuncture Mechanisms of Pain Modulation," in G. Stux and R. Hammershlag, eds., *Clinical Acupuncture, Scientific Basis* (Berlin and Heidelberg: Springer, 2001), 51-68. For evidence of another analgesic mechanism, see Nanna Goldman et al., "Adenosine A1 Receptors Mediate Local Anti-Nociceptive Effects of Acupuncture," *Nature Neuroscience*, 13, no. 7 (2010): 883-888.

34. Gabriel Stux, Brian Berman, and Bruce Pomeranz, *Basics of Acupuncture* (New York: Springer, 1988), 8-21, esp. 14. Despite the strong evidence for the endogenous opioid theory, Pomeranz stated "there's more to acupuncture than endogenous opioids. I'm not claiming this is all of it. I'm just claiming a small part of it." In "Bruce Pomeranz, PhD. Acupuncture and the Raison d'Être for Alternative Medicine. Interview by Bonnie Horrigan," *Alternative Therapies in Health and Medicine* (November 1996), 2, no. 6, 85-91.

35. Ted J. Kaptchuk, *The Web That Has No Weaver: Understanding Chinese Medicine* (New York: McGraw-Hill, 2000), 21.

36. These observations come from the author's experience in research, discussions at conferences and journal clubs, and personal conversations with researchers from 2012 to 2020.

37. See for example Claudia Witt et al., "Acupuncture in Patients with Osteoarthritis of the Knee: A Randomised Trial," *Lancet*, 366 (2005): 136-143; Michael Haake et al., "German Acupuncture Trials (GERAC) for Chronic Low Back Pain," *Archives of Internal Medicine*, 167, no. 17 (2007): 1892-1898; Andrew J. Vickers et al., "Acupuncture for Chronic Pain: Individual Patient Data Meta-analysis," *Archives of Internal Medicine*, 172, no. 19 (2012): 1444-1453.

38. Steven Birch, "Reflections on the German Acupuncture Studies," *Journal of Chinese Medicine*, no. 83 (2007): 12-17.

39. Haake et al., "German Acupuncture Trials," 1898.

40. Ibid., 1896.

41. Usual care is a nonspecific term that includes a range of options that might be offered to the patient; the patient has a choice to accept or not. The idea is that usual care represents what the patient would be doing for their condition if not undergoing the trial therapy.

42. The topic became one of intense discussion; see Helene M. Langevin et al., "Paradoxes in Acupuncture Research: Strategies for Moving Forward," *Evidence-Based Complementary and Alternative Medicine* (2011): doi: 10.1155/2011/180805; Ted J. Kaptchuk, Chen Ke-Ji, & Song Jun, "Recent Trials of Acupuncture in the West: Responses from Practitioners," *Chinese Journal of Integrative Medicine*, 16, no. 3 (2010): 197-203, doi: 10.1007/s11655-010-0197-x.

43. Congress renamed the NCCAM the National Center for Complementary and Integrative Health (NCCIH) in December 2014.

44. Kaptchuk was speaking at the 2018 Pacific Symposium in San Diego, an annual conference on acupuncture and Chinese medicine, which is the largest of its kind in the United States. The author was in attendance. Kaptchuk described how the NIH brought in leading acupuncturists and methodologists from across the United States and Europe to develop a study that would demonstrate acupuncture is more than placebo. According to Kaptchuk, he was invited but declined to participate in the study as he did not think the methodology would produce valid results.

45. Daniel C. Cherkin et al., "A Randomized Trial Comparing Acupuncture, Simulated Acupuncture, and Usual Care for Chronic Low Back Pain," *Archives of Internal Medicine*, 169, no. 9 (2009): 858-866, doi: 10.1001/archinternmed.2009.65.

46. Ted J. Kaptchuk et al., "Components of Placebo Effect: Randomised Controlled Trial in Patients with Irritable Bowel Syndrome," *BMJ*, 336, no. 7651 (2008): 999-1003, doi: 10.1136/bmj.39524.439618.25. The supportive patient/practitioner interaction included warmth, active listening, meaningful touch (pulse-taking), 20 seconds of thoughtful silence during the pulse-taking, and expressions of confidence and expectation for positive treatment results by the practitioner.

47. Ted J. Kaptchuk et al., "Placebos without Deception: A Randomized Controlled Trial in Irritable Bowel Syndrome," *PLoS One*, 5, no. 12 (2010): doi: 10.1371/journal.pone.0015591.

48. Kaptchuk, 2018 Pacific Symposium.

49. The contentious debate around using sham controls in acupuncture trials arose largely because the conventional standard for acceptance of a new treatment in biomedicine is evidence that the treatment's effect is greater than the placebo effect. The standard was designed to test the efficacy of pharmaceutical drugs, however, not complex whole-systems interventions. For a critical discussion, see Charlotte Paterson and Paul Dieppe, "Characteristic and Incidental (Placebo) Effects in Complex Interventions Such as Acupuncture," *BMJ*, 330, no. 7501 (2005): 1202-1205, doi: 10.1136/bmj.330.7501.1202.

50. Hugh MacPherson, "Towards a Better Understanding of Why So Many Acupuncture Trials are 'Negative' in Contrast to Results Often Seen in Clinical Practice," 2nd International Symposium on Research in Acupuncture, Bologna, Italy, October 21, 2018. The author was in attendance.

51. Vickers et al., "Acupuncture for Chronic Pain," 1444-1453.

52. Ibid., 1444. The work was also funded by a grant from the Samueli Institute, while two British researchers were funded partially or entirely by the United Kingdom's National Institute for Health Research.

53. Yumi Maeda et al., "Rewiring the Primary Somatosensory Cortex in Carpal Tunnel Syndrome with Acupuncture," *Brain*, 140, no. 4 (2017): 914-927, doi: 10.1093/brain/awx015.

54. Cassidy, "Chinese Medicine Users in the United States, Part I," 22.

55. C. M. Cassidy, "Chinese Medicine Users in the United States, Part II: Preferred Aspects of Care," *Journal of Alternative and Complementary Medicine*, 4, no. 2 (1998): 189-202.

56. Charlotte Paterson and Nicky Britten, "Acupuncture for People with Chronic Illness: Combining Qualitative and Quantitative Outcome

Assessment," *Journal of Alternative and Complementary Medicine*, 9, no. 5 (2003): 671-681, doi: 10.1089/107555303322524526.

57. Ibid., 674.

58. Charlotte Paterson and Nicky Britten, "The Patient's Experience of Holistic Care: Insights from Acupuncture Research," *Chronic Illness*, 4 (2008): 264:277, doi: 10.1177/1742395308100648. The findings suggest that acupuncture in a clinical research context is suboptimal, another reason it might struggle to outperform sham techniques in clinical trials.

59. Ibid., 275.

60. Ted Kaptchuk, "Placebo Studies and Ritual Therapy: A Comparative Analysis of Navajo, Acupuncture, and Biomedical Healing," *Philosophical Transactions of the Royal Society of Medicine. Series B, Biological Sciences*, 366, no. 1572 (2011): 1849-1858, doi: 10.1098/rstb.2010.0385.

61. The terms "ear acupuncture" and "auricular acupuncture" are often used interchangeably. Andreas Wirz-Ridolfi, a medical doctor and scholar of auricular medicine, distinguishes between "ear acupuncture" ("a general term describing all diagnostic and therapeutic measures using points on the ear") and "auriculotherapy," which refers to the French school of ear acupuncture that sprang from the physician Paul Nogier. Wirz-Ridolfi prefers a term coined by Nogier himself—"auriculomedicine"— spanning "a whole complete and independent branch of medical science." See Andreas Wirz-Ridolfi, "The History of Ear Acupuncture and Ear Cartography: Why Precise Mapping of Auricular Points Is Important," *Medical Acupuncture*, 31, no. 3 (2019): 145-156, http://doi.org/10.1089/acu.2019.1349.

62. Linda L. Barnes, "A World of Chinese Medicine and Healing: Part One," in *Chinese Medicine and Healing: An Illustrated History*, eds. T. J. Hinrichs and Linda L. Barnes (Cambridge, MA: The Belknap Press of Harvard University Press, 2013), 290-292.

63. Ibid., 291-292.

64. Hsu, "Innovations in Acumoxa," 427-429.

65. Ibid., 422.

66. Ibid., 428. Hsu adds that, while ear acupuncture is used in Europe, "it remains in the realm of the bizarre" [as of the mid-1990s].

## CHAPTER 3 NOTES

1.  Michael Smith at Working Class Acupuncture October Revolution Conference, October 25, 2009, https://www.youtube.com/watch?v=4vebo0lQqQ4.

2.  Franklin Apfel, email communication with the author, May 1, 2019

3.  Barbara Zeller, telephone interview with the author, April 19, 2019; MBGC. Zeller mentioned the ZANU ambulance benefit, which was advertised in a poster created by the MBGC.

4.  Michael Glenn, "Introduction," in *The Radical Therapist: The Radical Therapist Collective*, ed. Jerome Agel (New York: Ballantine Books, 1971), xi.

5.  "Manifesto," in *The Radical Therapist*, xv-xxiii; Michael Glenn, "On Training Therapists," in *The Radical Therapist*, 8-17.

6.  James Doucet-Battle, *Sweetness in the Blood: Race, Risk, and Type 2 Diabetes* (Minneapolis: University of Minnesota Press, 2021), 94.

7.  Rodd Aya et al., *The Opium Trail: Heroin and Imperialism* (Somerville, MA: New England Free Press, April 1972), 81.

8.  Walter Bosque, speaking on a panel at the Colegio de Abogados in San Juan, Puerto Rico, headed "Salud, Dignidad, y Pobreza: Un Asunto de Derechos Humanos" ("Health, Dignity, and Poverty: A Matter of Human Rights"). Attended by the author on April 18, 2018.

9.  Franklin Apfel, telephone interview with the author, May 27, 2019.

10. Ibid.

11. Carlos Alvarez was speaking at a public memorial service for Michael Smith at the New York Society for Ethical Culture in New York. Attended by the author on March 24, 2018.

12. Aya et al., *The Opium Trail*, 80.

13. Alvarez, speaking at the public memorial service for Michael Smith.

14. Debbie Smith, Michael Smith's ex-wife, speaking at the public memorial service for Michael Smith.

15. Debbie Smith and Jeannette Robinson, Michael Smith's administrative assistant, speaking at the public memorial service for Michael Smith.

16. Anne Lown, telephone interview with the author, April 11, 2019; Jeannette Robinson, speaking at the public memorial service for Michael Smith.

17. Debbie Smith, speaking at the public memorial service for Michael Smith.

18. Interview with Mutulu Shakur in "RBG-Dr Mutulu Shakur, Healer of the People 1," YouTube video, 11:07, posted by New Afrikan Independence Movement, June 17, 2012, https://www.youtube.com/watch?v=4F7bwCJb_xs.

19. The Ocean Hill-Brownsville controversy was part of a wider experiment including three school districts. Inspired by parental concerns over failing schools, it tried to decentralize school governance from the bureaucracy-bogged Board of Education. The experiment caused an uproar after 19 teachers and supervisors, all white, were transferred out of the district. The teachers' union revolted; resulting strikes closed schools for much of the fall 1968 semester. For a deeper discussion, see Charles S. Isaacs, *Inside Ocean Hill-Brownsville: A Teacher's Education, 1968-1969* (Albany: State University of New York Press, 2014) and Diane Ravitch, *The Great School Wars: A History of the New York City Public Schools* (Baltimore: Johns Hopkins University Press, 1974).

20. Shakur, "RBG-Healer of the People 1" interview.

21. Ibid.

22. Ibid.

23. Jackie Haught, telephone interview with the author, May 5, 2019.

24. Shakur, "RBG-Healer of the People 1" interview.

25. Apfel, interview.

26. Bosque, speaking at the Colegio de Abogados.

27. Apfel, interview.

28. Ibid.

29. Tatsuo Hirano, telephone interview with the author, August 15, 2020.

30. "2018 Interview about Acupuncture & the Opioid Crisis," interview by Olga Khazan, Mutulu Shakur, November 19, 2018, http://mutulushakur.com/site/2018/11/acupuncture-interview/.

31. Ibid.

32. Bosque, speaking at the Colegio de Abogados.

33. *Dope is Death*, directed by Mia Donovan (Toronto: EyeSteelFilm, 2020), film.

34. Apfel, interview.

35. "Oriental" was the commonly used modifier to describe Chinese medicine when acupuncture first gained popularity in the United States. It made its way into the names of many acupuncture colleges and associations. The

term is now recognized as derogatory; "Chinese medicine" is accepted but some prefer the term "East Asian medicine" to acknowledge the contributions of other regions, including Japan and Vietnam (formerly as part of Indochina) where the medicine was developed. The word "oriental" will only be used as part of proper nouns or in quotation marks to designate its past usage in this book.

36. Tamara Venit Shelton, *Herbs and Roots: A History of Chinese Doctors in the American Medical Marketplace* (New Haven: Yale University Press, 2019), 245.

37. Apfel, interview.

38. H. L. Wen and S. Y. C. Cheung. "Treatment of Drug Addiction by Acupuncture and Electrical Stimulation," *Asian Medicine Journal*, 9 (1973): 138–141.

39. Apfel, interview.

40. White Lightning, "People's Doctor Murdered! … an unsuccessful attempt to destroy the Lincoln Detox drug program" (Bronx, NY: Done at Come! Unity Press [undated]), https://www.freedomarchives.org/Documents/Finder/DOC58_scans/58.White.Lightening.RichardTaft.pdf.

41. Apfel, interview.

42. Ibid. While Apfel recalled knowing Taft through Columbia, Taft is reported to have graduated from Baylor College of Medicine in Houston.

43. "Doctor's Body Found at Hospital," *Daily News*, news briefs, October 30, 1974.

44. Richard Severo, "Lyndon LaRouche, Cult Figure Who Ran for President 8 Times, Dies at 96," *New York Times*, February 13, 2019, https://www.nytimes.com/2019/02/13/obituaries/lyndon-larouche-dead.html.

45. The furious accusations appeared in two publications released after Taft's death: "Terror Erupts at Lincoln Detox," EIR, 1, no. 28, EIR News Service, Inc., October 30, 1974; and White Lightning, "People's Doctor Murdered" [undated].

46. Shakur, "2018 Interview about Acupuncture & the Opioid Crisis."

47. Ward Churchill and Jim Vander Wall, *The COINTELPRO Papers* (Boston: South End Press, 1990), 110. The raid, which had been facilitated by an informant, was launched by a 14-man police team at around 4 o'clock in the morning. Thirteen years later, survivors were awarded $1.85 million in damages. Martin Luther King, Jr.—who was assassinated the month after the memo—Nation of Islam leader Elijah Muhammad, and Stokely Carmichael, the charismatic speaker who has been credited with coining

the term "Black Power," were named as contenders to be "a real threat in this way."

48. John Castelluci, *The Big Dance: The Untold Story of Weatherman Kathy Boudin and the Terrorist Family that Committed the Brink's Robbery Murders* (New York: Dodd, Mead & Company, 1986), 73.

49. Michael Smith at Working Class Acupuncture October Revolution Conference.

50. Ibid.

51. Ibid.; Shakur, "2018 Interview about Acupuncture & the Opioid Crisis."

52. Shakur, "2018 Interview about Acupuncture & the Opioid Crisis." The Weather Underground Organization (initially the Weatherman, after Bob Dylan's lyric, "You don't need a weatherman to know which way the wind blows") was an offshoot of SDS. Its rhetoric, and sometimes active violence, in the name of revolution resulted in intense targeting by the FBI. The May 19th Communist Organization and its relative, the MBGC, evolved from the Weather Underground.

53. Zeller, interview.

54. Hirano, interview.

55. Misha Cohen, telephone interview with the author, December 8, 2019.

56. Ibid.

57. Hirano, interview.

58. Ibid.

59. Cohen, interview.

60. Shakur, "2018 Interview about Acupuncture & the Opioid Crisis."

61. Ibid.

62. Zeller, interview.

63. Cohen, interview.

64. Haught, interview.

65. Ibid.

66. Cohen, interview.

67. Ibid.

68. Hirano, interview.

69. Haught, interview.

70. Ibid.

71. The college was later named Institut de Médicine Traditionelle Chinoise du Montreal but has since closed.

72. Linda L. Barnes, "A World of Chinese Medicine and Healing: Part One," in T. J. Hinrichs and Linda L. Barnes, eds., *Chinese Medicine and Healing: An Illustrated History* (Cambridge, MA: The Belknap Press of Harvard University Press, 2013), 296.

73. Mario Wexu was speaking at the panel discussion at the Colegio de Abogados in San Juan, Puerto Rico, headed, "Salud, Dignidad, y Pobreza: Un Asunto de Derechos Humanos" ("Health, Dignity, and Poverty: A Matter of Human Rights"). Attended by the author on April 18, 2018.

74. Mario Wexu, "Dr. Mario Wexu and Amrit Singh 2/2," YouTube video, 5:17, posted by Six Degrees Community Acupuncture, April 4, 2016, https://www.youtube.com/watch?v=F9nUUkqBqw0.

75. Ibid.

76. Haught, interview; Cohen, interview.

77. Zeller, interview. Zeller remembered the Wexus as "very anti-doctor" because of the medical profession's effort, in Canada as in the United States, to exclude non-MDs from the practice of acupuncture. She cited a lack of respect for the science, history, and tradition of acupuncture as contributing to the professional bias against it.

78. Mutulu Shakur and Michael Smith, "The Use of Acupuncture in the Treatment of Drug Addiction," *American Journal of Acupuncture*, 7, no. 3 (July-September 1979): 223-228.

79. Shakur, "2018 Interview about Acupuncture & the Opioid Crisis."

80. Ronald Sullivan, "Countercharges by Lincoln Drug Unit," *New York Times*, November 30, 1978, https://www.nytimes.com/1978/11/30/archives/countercharges-by-lincoln-drug-unit-fear-of-disturbance-eases.html.

81. Bosque, speaking at the Colegio de Abogados.

82. Shakur, "2018 Interview about Acupuncture & the Opioid Crisis."

83. Bosque, speaking at the Colegio de Abogados, and Sullivan, "Countercharges by Lincoln Drug Unit."

## CHAPTER 4 NOTES

1.  The neighborhood—officially named the St. Nicholas Historic District in 1967—is a clearly delineated four blocks of homes built in the 1890s as a high-end development to sell to the white elite of Manhattan. The plan fell apart due to financial difficulties and changing demographics, and the homes were finally sold to African Americans at the price of $8,000 apiece. By the 1930s, the blocks were home to Black artists, musicians, and professionals and so earned the designation of Strivers Row. See Kelli Trapnell, "History of NYC Streets: Strivers Row," *Untapped New York*, last modified December 20, 2012, https://untappedcities.com/2012/12/20/history-of-streets-strivers-row/.

2.  Jackie Haught, telephone interview with the author, May 5, 2019.

3.  Karen Cutler, telephone interviews with the author, April 12, 2019, and August 3, 2019. Cutler noted that lectures at the acupuncture college she attended in California were often given in Chinese and translated to English. The five elements or five phases are an important part of classical Chinese medicine theory that appear in the earliest texts. Five-element theory is based on the ancient Chinese world view that human physiology is a microcosm of the universal laws of nature and is the foundation for the concept of yin/yang. J. R. Worsley (1923-2003), a British acupuncturist and educator, developed a modern school known as Five-Element Acupuncture.

4.  Cutler, interview.

5.  Haught, interview.

6.  Barbara Zeller, telephone interview with the author, April 19, 2019.

7.  Cutler, interview.

8.  Mutulu Shakur, "Honoring Urayoana Trinidad, Acupuncturist," posted on May 4, 1999, http://mutulushakur.com/site/1999/05/honoring-urayoana-trinidad/.

9.  Anne Lown, telephone interview with the author, April 16, 2019.

10. Mary Patten, *Revolution as an Eternal Dream: The Exemplary Failure of the Madame Binh Graphics Collective* (Chicago: Half Letter Press LLC, 2011), 11.

11. Ibid., 30-33.

12. Ibid., 30.

13. Fitzhugh Mullan, *White Coat, Clenched Fist: The Political Education of an American Physician* (Ann Arbor: University of Michigan Press, 1976, 2006), 194-197.

14. Patten, *Revolution as an Eternal Dream*, 49.

15. Interview with Mutulu Shakur in "RBG-Dr Mutulu Shakur, Healer of the People 1," YouTube video, 11:07, posted by New Afrikan Independence Movement, June 17, 2012, https://www.youtube.com/watch?v=4F7bwCJb_xs.

16. "National Task Force for COINTELPRO Litigation and Research," published by the National Task Force for COINTELPRO Litigation and Research, 1978, in the Freedom Archives, http://freedomarchives.org/Documents/Finder/DOC510_scans/COINTELPRO/510.COINTELPRO.NationalTaskforceCOINTELPRO.statement.pdf.

17. Cutler, interview.

18. Patten, *Revolution as an Eternal Dream*, 51.

19. John Castellucci, "Informants in Key Role for U.S. Brink's Case," *Sunday Journal-News* (White Plains, NY), April 3, 1983.

20. Similarly, the parents of rapper Tupac Shakur took the names Afeni Shakur and Lumumba Shakur. Both were jailed as members of the Panther 21. Mutulu Shakur later became stepfather to Tupac.

21. Cutler, interview.

22. Haught, interview.

23. Patten, *Revolution as an Eternal Dream*, 51.

24. John Castellucci, "Clinic Staffers to Fight Brink's Case Subpoenas," *The Journal News* (White Plains, NY), April 8, 1982.

25. John Castellucci, "Informant Tells Court of Training for Brink's Heist," *The Journal-News* (White Plains, NY), June 9, 1983.

26. Ibid.

27. John Castellucci, "Brink's supporters vow to 'raise hell' here," *The Journal-News* (White Plains, NY), September 3, 1982.

28. Ibid.

29. Sigrid Schmalzer, Daniel S. Chard, and Alyssa Botelho, eds., *Science for the People: Documents from America's Movement of Radical Scientists* (Amherst: University of Massachusetts Press, 2018), 4.

30. Institute of Traditional Chinese Medicine of New York City course catalog (undated), 1. Provided to the author by Jackie Haught.

31. Ibid., 1.

32. Ibid., 2.

33. Ibid.

34. The concept of a degree in service of underserved communities began with BAAANA; when Tatsuo Hirano was awarded his degree for Doctor of Acupuncture in Traditional Chinese Medicine from BAAANA, he also received a special citation for "six years of social health service in underserved communities in North America." Tatsuo Hirano, telephone interview with the author, August 15, 2020.

35. For a full history of Alan Berkman's revolutionary activities, and subsequent rise as a global public health expert and champion among HIV/AIDS activists, see Susan M. Reverby, *Co-Conspirator for Justice: The Revolutionary Life of Dr. Alan Berkman* (Chapel Hill: The University of North Carolina Press, 2020).

36. Haught, interview.

37. Lown, interview.

38. Cutler, interview.

39. Lown, interview.

40. Ted J. Kaptchuk, *The Web That Has No Weaver: Understanding Chinese Medicine* (New York: McGraw-Hill, 2000). Kaptchuk was named Assistant Professor of Medicine at Harvard Medical School in 1998, became a full Professor of Medicine in 2013, and was appointed Professor of Global Health and Social Medicine in 2015. He also directs the Program in Placebo Studies and the Therapeutic Encounter at Beth Israel Deaconess Medical Center and Harvard Medical School.

41. Ted Kaptchuk, email communication with the author, February 27, 2020.

42. Ibid.

43. Ibid.

44. Lown, interview.

45. Haught, interview.

46. *Shakur v. Shinn*, "First Amended Complaint for Declaratory and Injunctive Relief," Case 5:18-cv-00628-SVW-AS, Document 20, filed August 21, 2018.

# CHAPTER 5 NOTES

1.  Peter Deadman, "Community Acupuncture—Making Ming Vases from Buckets: A Reply to Lisa Rohleder," *JCM*, no. 99, June 2012: 55-59.

2.  Lisa Rohleder, "Community Acupuncture: Making Buckets from Ming Vases," *JCM*, no. 98, February 2012: 22-25.

3.  Lisa Rohleder, interview with the author, Portland, OR, May 31, 2018.

4.  Lisa Rohleder, "Acupuncture and Social Entrepreneurship," *Acupuncture Today*, March 2006, vol. 7, issue 3.

5.  Lisa Rohleder, "Widening the Door: Privilege and Access," *Acupuncture Today*, January 2007, vol. 8, issue 1.

6.  "Chinoiserie," *Encyclopaedia Britannica*, https://www.britannica.com/art/chinoiserie; Tyler Phan, "American Chinese Medicine" (PhD diss., University College London, 2017), https://discovery.ucl.ac.uk/id/eprint/1571107/, 31-32.

7.  Hans Christian-Andersen, "The Emperor's New Clothes," *Andersen's Fairy Tales*, first published 1837.

8.  Rohleder, "Making Buckets from Ming Vases," 23.

9.  Deadman, "A Reply to Lisa Rohleder," 57.

10. Carolyn Reuben, "The History of NADA," http://carolynreuben.com/history-of-nada/.

11. Lisa Rohleder, *Acupuncture Points Are Holes: A Case Study in Social Entrepreneurship* (Portland, OR: POCA, 2017), 52.

12. Ibid., 55.

13. Ibid., 114.

14. Lisa Rohleder, personal communication with the author, Portland, OR, July 6, 2019.

15. Kory Ward-Cook, Susan A. Chapman, and Adam Burke, "A National Practice Analysis of Traditional East Asian Medicine," presented at the American Public Health Association annual meeting, San Diego, CA, 2008.

16. Lisa Achilles was speaking on a panel at "Liberation Acupuncture and Community Based Integrative Medicine: A POCA Tech Fundraiser Sponsored by CareOregon," in Portland, OR. Attended by the author on June 1, 2018.

17. "Timeline of the Movement," POCA Tech, http://pocatech.org/timeline-of-the-movement.

18. Lisa Rohleder et al., *The Little Red Book of Community Acupuncture, No. 3*, ed. Andy Wegman (Portland, OR: POCA, 2011), 20.

19. "Sociocratic Principles and Methods," The Center for Dynamic Community Governance, http://www.dynamic-governance.org/library/resource-library/sociocratic-principles-methods/.

20. "Liberation Acupuncture and Community Based Integrative Medicine," June 1, 2018.

21. Ibid.

22. Cris Monteiro, personal communication with the author, June 1, 2018.

23. For a narrative explanation of hot-spotting, see Atul Gawande, "The Hot Spotters: Can We Lower Medical Costs by Giving the Neediest Patients Better Care?" *New Yorker*, January 24, 2011.

24. Rohleder, speaking at "Liberation Acupuncture and Community Based Integrative Medicine," June 1, 2018.

25. Ibid.

26. Ibid.

27. Lisa Rohleder, "What I'm Learning in Acupuncture School," https://liberationacupuncture.org/node/85.

28. Miguel "Mickey" Melendez, *We Took the Streets: Fighting for Latino Rights with the Young Lords* (New York: St. Martin's Press, 2003), 120. Mullan describes HRUM members reading William Hinton's *Fanshen* and Edgar Snow's *Red Star Over China*, and works on the American labor movement, along with Mao's *Quotations from Chairman Mao Tse-Tung* (AKA the *Little Red Book*). See Fitzhugh Mullan, *White Coat, Clenched Fist: The Political Education of an American Physician* (Ann Arbor: University of Michigan Press, 1976, 2006).

29. "Liberation Psychology," Society for Community Research and Action, https://www.scra27.org/what-we-do/what-community-psychology/liberation-psychology/.

30. Liberation Acupuncture, "What is Liberation Acupuncture?" https://liberationacupuncture.org/.

31. Lisa Rohleder, "Liberation Acupuncture Backstory," via email communication with the author, July 7, 2019.

32. Rohleder, interview.

33. Ibid.

34. "Re: Comments on the Notice of Proposed Rulemaking on Gainful Employment," ACAOM, letter to US Department of Education, Docket Number: ED-2014-OPE-0039, May 23, 2014.

35. Amanda Gaitaud, "Stories of Struggle and Success: Looking at the Burden of Debt," *Acupuncture Today*, March 2018, vol. 19, issue 3.

36. "Position Paper Part 3: Retaliation," comment posted January 12, 2018, https://www.pocacoop.com/prick-prod-provoke/post/position-paper-part-3-retaliation.

37. Rohleder, personal communication.

38. Maslow's "Hierarchy of Needs" is presented as a pyramid with basic physical needs on the bottom, emotional/psychological needs in the middle, and self-actualization needs at the top. The lower needs must be met before the higher needs can be achieved. Abraham Maslow, "A Theory of Human Motivation," *Psychological Review*, 50, no. 4 (1943): 370–396, https://doi.org/10.1037/h0054346.

39. Skip Van Meter lecture at POCA Tech, Portland, OR, July 6, 2019. The author was in attendance.

40. Ibid.

41. Rohleder, "Liberation Acupuncture Backstory."

42. Lisa Rohleder, email communication with the author, December 8, 2019.

43. Phan, "American Chinese Medicine," 3.

44. Edward W. Said, *Orientalism* (New York: Vintage Books, 1979; originally published by Pantheon Books, 1978); Rachel Adams, "Michel Foucault, Biopolitics and Biopower," *Critical Legal Thinking*, http://criticallegalthinking.com/2017/05/10/michel-foucault-biopolitics-biopower/.

45. James Reston, "Now About My Operation in Peking," *New York Times*, July 26, 1971, https://www.nytimes.com/1971/07/26/archives/now-about-my-operation-in-peking-now-let-me-tell-you-about-my.html. Reston's famous article, describing his experience with postappendectomy acupuncture while accompanying Henry Kissinger in China, is frequently attributed with having ignited American interest in acupuncture.

46. As quoted in Phan, "American Chinese Medicine," 82.

47. Ironically, the AMA is the very organization the radical medical students of the late 1960s sought to counter with the SHO.

48. Phan, "American Chinese Medicine," 88.

49. Phan was speaking at a POCAfest workshop headlined, "Understanding and Dismantling Systemic Oppression as Community Acupuncturists," at Crieff Hills in Ontario, Canada. Attended by the author on August 11, 2018.

50. Rohleder, email communication.

51. Ibid.

## CHAPTER 6 NOTES

1. Sigrid Schmalzer, Daniel S. Chard, and Alyssa Botelho, eds., *Science for the People: Documents from America's Movement of Radical Scientists* (Amherst: University of Massachusetts Press, 2018).

2. Ibid., 5.

3. Johanna Fernández, *The Young Lords: A Radical History* (Chapel Hill: University of North Carolina Press, 2020), 222.

4. Susan M. Reverby, interviewed by the author in "Co-Conspirator for Justice: The Revolutionary Life of Dr. Alan Berkman," November 27, 2020, in *New Books Network*, podcast, 0:40.22. https://newbooksnetwork.com/co-conspirator-for-justice.

5. Fernández, *The Young Lords*, 376-377; Reverby, *Co-Conspirator for Justice: The Revolutionary Life of Dr. Alan Berkman* (Chapel Hill: University of North Carolina Press, 2020), 124. Reverby writes that radicals endeavored to lead a revolution without realizing that no one was following them.

6. Reverby, *Co-Conspirator for Justice*, 114.

7. Ibid., 108.

8. For an excellent analysis of problems and solutions surrounding the aging of incarcerated people, see Tina Maschi and Keith Morgen, *Aging behind Prison Walls: Studies in Trauma and Resilience* (New York: Columbia University Press, 2020).

9. Mutulu Shakur, "Towards a Truth and Reconciliation Commission for New African/Black Political Prisoners, Prisoners of War and Freedom Fighters," May 5, 2010, http://mutulushakur.com/site/2010/05/trc-for-new-african-political-prisoners/.

10. As most graduates will go into private practice, US acupuncture colleges expect them to be able to grow a profitable business. In pursuit of this goal, students may be encouraged to pursue a wealthy clientele and set high prices. In one practice management class, students were advised

to imagine how much money they wanted to make and even what they would buy with it. At the same time, I have heard college administration minimize the usefulness of offsite clinics for underserved populations as it was claimed students would not be involved in such clinics after graduation. The reasons given were the lack of prestige in working at a low- or no-cost clinic outside of a biomedical institution and the need for graduates to earn enough to pay off student loans. High tuition and the heavy dependence of both colleges and students on federal financial aid certainly are disincentives to working with populations in need, according to my informal conversations with students and colleagues. For more insight into the dynamics of US acupuncture education, see Tyler Phan, "American Chinese Medicine" (PhD diss., University College London, 2017), https://discovery.ucl.ac.uk/id/eprint/1571107/.

11. In 2021, POCA updated its mission and vision statement to include "Work with regulators to ease entry into the acupuncture profession and engage with legislative processes to ensure safety and access are prioritized."

12. Susan Rosenberg, *An American Radical: Political Prisoner in My Own Country* (New York: Citadel Press, 2011), 24-25.

13. Jackie Haught, telephone interview with the author, May 5, 2019.

14. Ibid.

15. Tatsuo Hirano, telephone interview with the author, August 15, 2020.

16. Lisa Rohleder, "What I'm Learning in Acupuncture School," Liberation Acupuncture website, https://liberationacupuncture.org/node/85.

17. "Acu-Points: Black Acupuncture Meet and Greet," hosted by Tenisha Dandridge, YouTube video, 1:14.31, posted August 11, 2020, https://www.youtube.com/watch?v=iRTLA9tuzyQ.

18. Hirano, interview.

19. David Woo, "Marcus Books, the Nation's Oldest Black Bookstore: Historical Essay," in Shaping San Francisco's Digital Archive @ Found SF, http://www.foundsf.org/index.php?title=Marcus_Books,_the_Nation%E2%80%99s_Oldest_Black_Bookstore; "Oakland's Marcus Books still thrives as nation's oldest Black bookstore," KTVU Fox 2, February 15, 2019, https://www.ktvu.com/news/oaklands-marcus-books-still-thrives-as-nations-marcus-books-still-Black-bookstore; Aria Danaparamita, "Marcus Books: Oldest African-American Bookstore Fights to Stay Open," in National Trust for Historic Preservation, August 13, 2013, https://savingplaces.org/stories/marcus-books-oldest-african-american-bookstore-fights-to-stay-open.

20. Felicia Parker-Rodgers, email communication with the author, December 18, 2019.

21. Yvonne Scarlett, email communication with the author, December 20, 2019.

22. Tenisha Dandridge, telephone interview with the author, June 30, 2020.

23. Monica Garcia, email communication with the author, January 8, 2020, and telephone interview with the author, January 14, 2020.

24. Garcia, interview.

## EPILOGUE NOTES

1. Sonia Lopez, telephone interview with the author, March 25, 2019.

2. Jeannette Robinson and Carlos Alvarez were speaking at Michael Smith's public memorial service at the New York Society for Ethical Culture, attended by the author on March 24, 2018.

3. Jackie Haught, telephone interview with the author, May 5, 2019.

4. Walter Bosque was speaking on a panel at the Colegio de Abogados in San Juan, Puerto Rico, headed "Salud, Dignidad, y Pobreza: Un Asunto de Derechos Humanos" ("Health, Dignity, and Poverty: A Matter of Human Rights"). Attended by the author on April 18, 2018.

5. Barbara Zeller, telephone interview with the author, April 19, 2019.

6. Michael Smith at Working Class Acupuncture October Revolution Conference, October 25, 2009, https://www.youtube.com/watch?v=4vebo0lQqQ4.

7. Ibid.

8. "2018 Interview about Acupuncture & the Opioid Crisis," interview by Olga Khazan, Mutulu Shakur, November 19, 2018, http://mutulushakur.com/site/2018/11/acupuncture-interview/.

9. Mark Kleiman, telephone interview with the author, July 4, 2020.

10. *Shakur v. Shinn*, "First Amended Complaint for Declaratory and Injunctive Relief," Case 5:18-cv-00628-SVW-AS, Document 20, filed August 21, 2018, 22.

# Bibliography

*A Barefoot Doctor's Manual: The American Translation of the Official Chinese Paramedical Manual*. Philadelphia, PA: Running Press, 1977.

Agel, Jerome, ed. *The Radical Therapist: The Radical Therapist Collective*. New York: Ballantine Books, 1971.

Ahmad, Muhammed (Maxwell Stanford, Jr.). *We Will Return in the Whirlwind: Black Radical Organizations 1960-1975*. Chicago, Charles H. Kerr Publishing Company, 2007.

Andrews, Bridie. *The Making of Modern Chinese Medicine, 1850-1960*. Honolulu: University of Hawaii Press, 2014.

Berman, Marshall. *All That Is Solid Melts into Air: The Experience of Modernity* (New York: Penguin Books, 1988).

Brazelton, Mary Augusta. *Mass Vaccination: Citizens' Bodies and State Power in Modern China*. Ithaca: Cornell University Press, 2019.

Caro, Robert A. *The Power Broker: Robert Moses and the Fall of New York*. New York: Vintage Books, 1974.

Castelluci, John. *The Big Dance: The Untold Story of Weatherman Kathy Boudin and the Terrorist Family that Committed the Brink's Robbery Murders*. New York: Dodd, Mead & Company, 1986.

Churchill, Ward and Jim Vander Wall. *The COINTELPRO Papers.* Boston: South End Press, 1990.

Crozier, Ralph C. *Traditional Medicine in Modern China.* Cambridge, MA: Harvard University Press; London: Oxford University Press, 1968.

Deadman, Peter and Mazin Al-Khafaji with Kevin Baker. *A Manual of Acupuncture.* East Sussex, England: Journal of Chinese Medicine Publications, 2007.

Ehrenreich, Barbara and John, eds. *The American Health Empire: Power, Profits and Politics. A Report from the Health Policy Advisory Center (Health/PAC).* New York: Vintage Books, 1970.

Elbaum, Max. *Revolution in the Air: Sixties Radicals Turn to Lenin, Mao, and Che.* New York: Verso, 2002, 2018.

Fang, Xiaoping. *China and the Cholera Pandemic: Restructuring Society under Mao.* Pittsburgh: University of Pittsburgh Press, 2021.

Fernández, Johanna. *The Young Lords: A Radical History.* Chapel Hill: University of North Carolina Press, 2020.

Hinrichs, T.J. and Linda L. Barnes, eds. *Chinese Medicine and Healing: An Illustrated History.* Cambridge, MA: The Belknap Press of Harvard University Press, 2013.

Hutchison, Alan. *China's African Revolution.* Boulder, CO: Westview Press, 1975.

Kaptchuk, Ted J. *The Web That Has No Weaver: Understanding Chinese Medicine.* New York: McGraw-Hill, 2000.

Kempton, Murray. *The Briar Patch: The People of the State of New York v. Lumumba Shakur et al.* New York: E.P. Dutton Co., Inc., 1973.

kioni-sadiki, déqui and Matt Meyer, eds. *Look for Me in the Whirlwind: From the Panther 21 to 21st-Century Revolutions.* Oakland, CA: PM Press, 2017.

Lee, Sun. "WHO and the developing world: the contest for ideology." In *Western Medicine as Contested Knowledge*, ed. by Andrew Cunningham and Bridie Andrews, 24-45. Manchester, UK: Manchester University Press, 1997.

Lei, Sean Hsiang-Lin. *Neither Donkey nor Horse: Medicine in the Struggle Over China's Modernity*. London: University of Chicago Press, 2014.

Lovell, Julia. *Maoism: A Global History*. New York: Alfred A. Knopf, 2019.

McCoy, Alfred W. with Catherine B. Read and Leonard P. Adams II. *The Politics of Heroin in Southeast Asia*. New York: Harper & Row, 1972.

Melendez, Miguel "Mickey." *We Took the Streets: Fighting for Latino Rights with the Young Lords*. New York: St. Martin's Press, 2003.

Mitchell, Ellinor R. *Fighting Drug Abuse with Acupuncture: The Treatment that Works*. Berkeley, CA: Pacific View Press, 1995.

Mullan, Fitzhugh. *White Coat, Clenched Fist: The Political Education of an American Physician*. Ann Arbor: University of Michigan Press, 1976, 2006.

Nelson, Alondra. *Body and Soul: The Black Panther Party and the Fight Against Medical Discrimination*. Minneapolis: University of Minnesota Press, 2011.

Patten, Mary. *Revolution as an Eternal Dream: The Exemplary Failure of the Madame Binh Graphics Collective*. Chicago: Half Letter Press LLC, 2011.

Pickowicz, Paul. *A Sensational Encounter with High Socialist China*. Hong Kong: City University of Hong Kong, 2019.

Reverby, Susan M. *Co-Conspirator for Justice: The Revolutionary Life of Dr. Alan Berkman*. Chapel Hill: University of North Carolina Press, 2020.

Risse, Guenter B., ed. *Modern China and Traditional Chinese Medicine*. Springfield, IL: Charles C. Thomas, Publisher, 1973.

Rohleder, Lisa. *Acupuncture Points Are Holes: A Case Study in Social Entrepreneurship*. Portland, OR: People's Organization of Community Acupuncture, 2017.

Rohleder, Lisa, Nora Madden, Larry Gatti, Jr., and Julia Carpenter. *The Little Red Book of Community Acupuncture, No. 3.*, ed. Andy Wegman. Portland, OR: People's Organization of Community Acupuncture, 2011.

Rosenberg, Susan. *An American Radical: Political Prisoner in My Own Country*. New York: Citadel Press, 2011.

Rosenthal, Mel. *In the South Bronx of America*. Willimantic, CT: Curbstone Press, 2000.

Roszak, Theodore. *The Making of a Counter Culture: Reflections on the Technocratic Society and its Youthful Opposition*. Garden City, NY: Anchor Books, 1969.

Said, Edward W. *Orientalism*. New York: Vintage Books, 1979; originally published by Pantheon Books, 1978.

Schmalzer, Sigrid, Daniel S. Chard, and Alyssa Botelho, eds. *Science for the People: Documents from America's Movement of Radical Scientists*. Amherst: University of Massachusetts Press, 2018.

Sidel, Victor W. and Ruth Sidel. *Serve the People: Observations on Medicine in the People's Republic of China*. New York: Josiah Macy, Jr. Foundation, 1973.

Smith, David E., David J. Bentel, and Jerome L. Schwartz, eds. *The Free Clinic: A Community Approach to Health Care and Drug Abuse*. Beloit, WI: Stash Press, 1971.

Stux, Gabriel, Brian Berman, and Bruce Pomeranz. *Basics of Acupuncture*. New York: Springer, 1988.

Taylor, Kim. *Chinese Medicine in Early Communist China, 1945-1963: A Medicine of Revolution*. London: Routledge, 2004.

Unschuld, Paul U. *Medicine in China: A History of Ideas*. Berkeley: University of California Press, 1985.

Veith, Ilza. *The Yellow Emperor's Classic of Internal Medicine, Translated, with an Introductory Study.* Berkeley: University of California Press, 1949, 1966.

Venit Shelton, Tamara. *Herbs and Roots: A History of Chinese Doctors in the American Medical Marketplace.* New Haven: Yale University Press, 2019.

Wallace, Deborah, and Rodrick Wallace. *A Plague on Your Houses: How New York Was Burned Down and National Public Health Crumbled.* New York: Verso, 1998.

Werner, David, David and Carol Thurman, and Jane Maxwell. *Where There Is No Doctor: A Village Health Care Handbook.* Berkeley, CA: Hesperian Health Guides, 1977.

Wiseman, Nigel and Andrew Ellis, eds. and trans. *Fundamentals of Chinese Medicine.* Brookline, MA: Paradigm Publications, 1996.

Zhan, Mei. *Other-Worldly: Making Chinese Medicine through Transnational Frames.* Durham: Duke University Press, 2009.

# Index

Abiodun, Nehanda, 184, 186

accreditation: Accreditation Commission for Acupuncture and Oriental Medicine (ACAOM), 68, 155, 158, 161; regulatory bodies for, 171

Achilles, Lisa, 149

acquired immunodeficiency syndrome (AIDS), 112, 137–39, 173–74

acupuncture: college, 12, 30, 32, 63, 68, 73, 98, 116–18, 123–24, 134, 145–46, 148, 155, 161, 170, 177, 182; countercultural influence, 25–26; drug abuse. *See* drug(s); global revolution and Maoism, 14–15; history, 7–10; media coverage, 17–22; perception and reception, 26–28; political vision, 124–25; qualitative research, 85–88; reemergence of, 77–79; regulation, 171; research, 79–82; scientization of, 72–74; traditional theory of, 112; *See also* barefoot doctor program

Acupuncture Advisory Board of Utah, 157

Acupuncture Coalition of New York, 133

Acupuncture Detox Specialists Collective, 176

*Acupuncture Today* (trade publication), 142, 149

Acupuncture Triallists Collaboration, 84–85

acupuncturists: activist, 9; Black, 176, 178, 182; Chinese, 26, 27; community, 9, 143–45, 151, 155–56, 160, 175, 177–78; criticism of, 144–45; distribution in the US, 68; French-Vietnamese, 116–17; in Chinatown, 100, 110; Latinx, 12, 32, 178; licensure, 68–72; Puerto Rican, 2–3; revolutionary, 9, 21, 29, 87, 90; training of, 69

Acupuncturists Without Borders (AWB), 2, 177

addiction: alcohol, 133–34, 146–47; drug(s), 49, 99, 112–13, 139, 165, 167, 168, 174, 176; heroin, 11–12, 38, 56–58, 62–63, 91, 102, 133–34; and methadone maintenance, 59–66; narcotics, role in colonialism, 63; opioid drug, 62–66, 103; in South Bronx, 59–66

Adolphene, 62

African Wholistic Health Association, 176

aging population in US prison system, 169
Albert Einstein College of Medicine, 19, 24, 44, 52
alcohol addiction. *See* addiction
alternative medicine, 7, 137
Alvarez, Carlos, 4, 95, 188
American Association of Acupuncture and Oriental Medicine, 133, 158
*American Journal of Acupuncture,* 119
American Medical Association (AMA), 44, 52, 63, 104
Andrews, Bridie, 78
Apfel, Franklin, 21–22, 55, 91, 93, 99, 102, 103, 104, 108, 110
*Asbury Park Press,* 18
Asian American activism, 28–29, 110
Asian Joint Communications, 110
auricular acupuncture, 30, 88–90, 101–2, 117, 123, 172

BAAANA (Black Acupuncture Advisory Association of North America), 30, 63, 160, 168–69, 171, 172, 175, 178, 182, 184, 186; Brink's robbery, 128–29, 130, 131, 134, 139, 168; Chinese medicine theory at, 135; and communication, other groups, 126; FBI raid, 128, 129; First World Acupuncture, 131, 132–39; forceful closure of, 131; formation, 121–22; closure by Joint Terrorist Task Force, 131; mix of motivations at, 127; operation, 122; political vision, 124–25; students, 124–25
Baldwin, James, 179
Baraldini, Silvia, 130
barefoot doctors: 23, 25, 69, 73, 134; activists' impression of, 21–22, 48–49, 111, 137; in Africa, 15–16; Chinese and Western media on, 17–22, 65, 100
Barke, Morton, 102
Barnes, Linda, 89
Bayer, 63
Bayete, Kamau (Peter Middleton), 130–31
Berkman, Alan, 109, 134, 169
Berman, Marshall, 36, 38
bias, 81, 155, 157, 162
biomedicine, 15, 26, 69–70, 72, 78, 81, 89
biopower, concept of, 162
Birch, Steven, 82
Black Liberation Army, 129
Black liberation movements, 14, 40, 55, 61, 107, 110, 115, 126–127, 128, 152, 165
Black militancy movements, 183–86
Black Panthers, 14, 15, 22, 26, 50, 61, 113, 115, 137, 168, 189
Black Power movement, 11, 12, 29, 58

Bosque, Walter, 34, 121, 188–89; and Lincoln Detox, 99–103, 109, 111, 115–17, 119–20
Bourne, Peter, 61
Bouza, Anthony, 40
BPP (Black Panther Party), 15, 22, 50, 95, 96, 126, 137, 154, 168, 184
Brazelton, Mary Augusta, 16, 28
Brink's robbery, 128–29, 130, 131, 134, 139, 168, 169, 184
Britten, Nicky, 87
Brody, Jane, 27
Bronx. *See* South Bronx
"The Bronx is Burning" (documentary series), 39
Bronx Legal Services Inc., 120
Brown, Waverly, 129
Buck, Marilyn, 138
Buddhism, 172, 173
Bu, Liping, 23
Burma, 57

California, legalization of acupuncture in, 73–74
CareOregon, 148–49, 150, 151
Caro, Robert, 36–37
carpal tunnel syndrome, 71, 85
Carter, Jimmy, 39
Cassidy, C. M., 86–87
Castro, Fidel, 15, 111
Centers for Disease Control and Prevention, 137
Central Intelligence Agency (CIA), 11, 56–58, 130
certification exams, NCCAOM, 157
Chamfrault, Albert, 89
chemical warfare, 11, 30, 56–59, 113, 114, 120, 121
chemotherapy-induced nausea, 71
Cheng Dan'an, 78–79
Chen Zhiqian, 23
Chesimard, Joanne, 129. *See also* Shakur, Assata
Cheung, S. Y. C., 103
China: and Africa, 8–9, 15; experience with opium addiction, 64–66; and Japan, 63, 78; and opium addiction, 64; and the US, 26–27; and the USSR, 15
Chinese Communist Party (CCP), 8, 15, 20
Chinese herbology, 69, 136, 157
Chinese medicine: accreditation at First World Acupuncture, 132; and auricular acupuncture, 89; correspondence course in, 102; dispute between Deadman and Rohleder, 145; immigrant practice and racism, 154; POCA Tech brief history, 159; holism, 49; and Horn, 65; Kaptchuk

degrees, acupuncture, 134; Black Acupuncture Advisory Association of North America, 122–23, 133; Chinese medicine, 137; Harlem Institute of Acupuncture, 122; master's degree, 157, 160, 178; NCCAOM exam, 157; Traditional Acupuncturist in Service to the Community, 134; without licensure, 118

Delaney, Richard, 109, 115–16, 117, 121, 122, 123, 129

Dellums, Ronald, 128

Designing Justice and Designing Spaces, 181–82

detox/detoxification, 60; Acupuncture Detox Specialists Collective, 176; branches of, 109–16; drug, 94, 169, 181; Hooper Detox, 146, 147; imprisonment for, 60; Lincoln Detox. *See* Lincoln Detox Acupuncture collective (Lincoln Detox); revolutionary detox acupuncture. *See* revolutionary detox acupuncture

diacetylmorphine, 63

dialectical materialism, 26, 76, 111

disposable needles, single-use, 138

Division of Occupational and Professional Licensing, 157

Dohrn, Bernardine, 109, 111

Dohrn, Jennifer, 109

Dolophine, 62

Doucet-Battle, James, 94

drug(s): acupuncture treatment for, 172, 181, 182, 189–90; addiction, 49, 99, 112–13, 139, 165, 167, 168, 174, 176; Bayete's testimony, 130–31; detoxification, method of, 94; detoxification and use, 168, 169; intravenous drug users, 138; multiple-drug abuse problems, 99–100; role, in community, 128; systemic use of, 125

ear acupuncture. *See* auricular acupuncture

education, acupuncture, 68–70; BAAANA. *See* BAAANA (Black Acupuncture Advisory Association of North America); cost, 157–58; First World Acupuncture, 131, 132–39, 170, 171; Pacific College of Health and Science, 177; POCA Tech. *See* POCA (People's Organization of Community Acupuncture); TCM. *See* TCM (Traditional Chinese Medicine)

Ehrenreich, Barbara, 44, 45

Einstein-Montefiore empire, 44–45

Eisen, David, 146

electroacupuncture, 74–75, 80

endogenous opioids, 80, 88

English, Joseph T., 55

ethnicity, 95, 102

Executive Intelligence Review (EIR) News Service, 106

expanded effects of care, 86

Haught, Jackie, 98, 112, 114, 115–16, 122, 124, 125, 129–30, 132, 134, 138, 172–73
Hay, Ing "Doc," 154
Health and Hospital Corporation, 54–55, 108, 119, 187
Health Policy Advisory Center (Health/PAC), 43–45, 50–51
Health Resilience program, 151, 152
Health Revolutionary Unity Movement (HRUM), 45, 46, 50, 52, 55
hepatitis B, 112
herbal medicine, 22, 24
herbology, Chinese, 69, 136, 157
1914 Heroin Narcotics Act, 62
Hirano, Tatsuo, 29, 110, 111, 114, 173, 176, 177
Hitler, Adolph, 62
Ho Chi Minh, 125
holism, 86, 87
holistic healthcare model, 86–87
Hooper, David, 146
Hooper Detox clinic, 146–47
Horn, Joshua S., 64–65, 100
hot-spotting, 151
Housing Act of 1949, 38
Hsu, Elisabeth, 74–75, 77–78, 89–90
human immunodeficiency virus (HIV), 112, 139

imprisonment for detoxification, 60
indigenous medicine, 9, 30, 48, 68, 88
Institute of National Medicine, 72–73, 78
Institute of Traditional Chinese Medicine of New York City, 131, 132
insurance, health, 112, 142, 152
International Association of Traditional Chinese Medicine, 133
International Justice Mission, 158
irritable bowel syndrome (IBS), placebo effects for, 83–84

Japan: and China, 63, 78; traditional medicine in, 78
Jewish immigrants, 32, 42
Johnson, Lyndon B., 39
Joint Committee of Physicians and Health Insurance Plans, 82
Joint Terrorist Task Force, 131, 171
*Journal of Chinese Medicine (JCM),* 141, 143, 155–56
*Journal of the American Medical Association,* 19
Jung Tao School of Classical Chinese Medicine in Sugar Grove, 69

Kampmann, Kate, 153

Macau Institute of Chinese Medicine, 137
MacPherson, Hugh, 84
Madame Binh Graphics Collective (MBGC), 92, 125, 126–27, 130, 154, 155
Malcolm X, 100, 125, 179
*Man Alive* (documentary), 39
Maoism, 11, 14–15, 25
Mao Zedong, 8, 15, 18, 47, 65–66, 103, 154
"Mao Zedong Thought" classes, 75, 76
Marcus Books, 178–80
Marti, José, 125
Martin-Baró, Ignacio, 154, 174
Maslow, Abraham, 159
May 19th Communist Organization, 125–27, 130, 134
McCoy, Alfred W., 56–58
McGee, Gale W., 58
Medicaid, 68, 148–49
medical diplomacy, 11, 15, 16, 18
medical doctors, 22, 31, 47–48, 52, 54, 70–71, 88, 108–9, 117–18, 120, 122, 163, 180, 187
Medicare, 68, 70–71
Meiji era, 78
Melendez, Miguel "Mickey," 33, 53, 64, 65, 120
Mendoza, Maria, 109
mental health services program, 45–48
Meo tribesman, 57, 58
methadone, 60, 62, 91, 133–34, 150; alternative therapy, 102; dispensation, 95; history, 117; maintenance, 94; overdose, 99; tapering, 93; treatment for detoxification, 100, 102
methadone maintenance, 60–66; development and promotion, 60–61; drawback of, 61
Middleton, Peter (Kamau Bayete), 130
Miyamoto, Nobuko, 29
modern Chinese medicine, 72, 76, 78
Monteiro, Cris, 151
Morant, George Soulié de, 88–89
morphine, 62–63
Morrison, Toni, 179
Moses, Robert, 36–37, 38
moxibustion, 27, 71–72
Moynihan, Daniel Patrick, 34
Mullan, Fitzhugh, 42–43, 50, 52, 53, 127
Murphy, Ricky, 109, 115–16, 117

NADA (National Acupuncture Detoxification Association), 120, 146, 147, 154, 169, 177, 187, 188

Napadow, Vitaly, 85

narcotics addiction and colonialism, 63–65

National Acupuncture Association, 162–63

National Association for the Advancement of Colored People (NAACP), 97

National Caucus of Labor Committees (NCLC), 106, 107

National Center for Complementary and Alternative Medicine (NCCAM), 83

National Commission for Certification of Acupuncture (NCCA) exam, 136, 138

National Drug Abuse Council, 108

National Institutes of Health (NIH), 82, 85

Nationalist Chinese guerrilla army, 57

National University, 68–69

Nazis, 116, 117; Nazi drug companies, 62

NCCAOM (National Certification Commission for Acupuncture and Oriental Medicine), 69, 157

Needham, Joseph, 77–78

needles: detox program without, 108; in ears, 103, 104, 111, 172; filiform, 78–79; marks, 104; placement of, 159, 172; points on body, 112; silver, 160; single-use disposable, 138; into sinus cavity of blind man, 116

needling, 22, 72, 74, 78, 138, 159, 172; adaptability to theoretical variation, 88; Chinese vs. Western, 81; "dry needling," 71; and placebo, 82; sham needling, 85

neurotransmitters, 80

*New England Journal of Medicine,* 19

New England School of Acupuncture, 137, 163

New Left, 11, 14–15, 58, 170

Newton, Huey, 22

New York Addiction Service Agency, 108

New York City-Rand Institute, 38–39

*New York Times,* 26–27, 55, 102, 103, 106, 162–63, 181

Nixon, Richard, 19, 34, 60, 100, 137

Nogier, Paul, 88, 89

Ocean Hill-Brownsville controversy, 97

O'Grady, Edward, 129

oncology acupuncture, 79, 85

opioid drug, 91; acupuncture therapy, 101; addiction, 62–65, 103; overdose, 99. *See also* drugs; methadone

Oregon College of Oriental Medicine (OCOM), 145, 146, 157

Orientalism, 143, 161–65

orientalization of American acupuncture, 161–65

Oriental medicine, 69, 102

Pacific College of Health and Science, 177, 178
Paige, Peter, 129
*Palante* (newspaper), 58
*Palm Beach Post-Times,* 17
Panther 21, 64–65
Parker-Rodgers, Felicia, 178–79, 183, 184
Parks, Rosa, 179
Paterson, Charlotte, 87
Patient Protection and Affordable Care Act in 2010, 67
Patten, Mary, 126–27
Patterson, Kokayi, 176
Peking Union Medical College (PUMC), 23, 27
people of color, 93, 95, 122, 173, 181
People's Program Court Collective, 103–4
Pericardium 6 (Neiguan or P6), 81
Phan, Tyler, 73–74, 161–62, 163–65, 182
Pickowicz, Paul, 75–76
placebo-controlled trials, 80–82
placebo effect, 82–85
POCA (People's Organization of Community Acupuncture), 134, 139, 177;
      CareOregon partnership, 148–49, 150, 151, 152; formation, 149; Health
      Resilience program, 151, 152; Liberation Acupuncture, 149, 152–56;
      mission, 149; overview, 141–45; POCAfests, 161, 163; POCA Tech, 12, 155,
      156–61, 164–65; POCAverse, 156; safe-space ethos, 150; Working Class
      Acupuncture, 145–49, 150, 151
*The Police Tapes* (documentary), 39
political prisoners, 94–95, 98, 124, 126, 127
Pomeranz, Bruce, 80
poverty, 24, 26, 36, 42, 49, 94, 143, 174, 176, 185; War on, 39
Prensky, William, 74
professional credentials, purpose of, 94
professionalism, 47–49; in community mental health workers, 94; Ding
      County experiment, 23–25; in licensed acupuncturists, 69–70, 118, 122;
      paternalistic hierarchy of, 100
Progressive Productions of Lincoln Detox Acupuncture, 92

Quebec Association of Acupuncture, 133
Quebec connection, 116–18
Quebec Institute of Acupuncture, 122

racism, 128, 178; anti-Asian, 28–29; anti-Black, 182–83; fight against, 94; George Floyd's killing, 177, 182–83; limits of political process for Black Americans, 97; medical doctors, 122; Patten on, 126–127; People's Organization of Community Acupuncture, members, 150; racist attacks, Ing "Doc" Hay, 154; Mutulu Shakur's perspective on, 128, 169

Racketeer Influenced and Corrupt Organizations (RICO) Act, 129, 138

radical movements, 130, 154, 155, 167, 168, 170

radicals: BAAANA. *See* BAAANA (Black Acupuncture Advisory Association of North America); Kaptchuk, 136–37, 163; Rohleder. *See* Rohleder, Lisa

*The Radical Therapist* (journal), 93, 94

Rand Corporation, 38

Red Guards, 136

Republic of New Afrika (RNA), 96, 98, 114, 115, 128

Reston, James, 26–27, 103, 162–63, 181

Reverby, Susan, 169

Revolutionary Armed Task Force, 129

revolutionary detox acupuncture, 93, 131, 165; and Asian American radical activism, 29; and barefoot doctors, 16, 21; beginning of, 11–12; branches of, 109–16; and chemical warfare, 59; and contemporary acupuncturists, 175–83; and countercultural ideologies, 26; Dandridge, 178, 181–83; and Ding County experiment, 23–25; Garcia, 183–86; and love, 172–73; Marcus Books, 178–80; origins of, 11–14; overview, 167–72; Scarlett, 180–81; and suffering, 172–73, 174–75

Robinson, Jeannette, 188

Rockefeller Foundation, 27

Rodriguez, Carmen, 96

Rohleder, Lisa, 141–43; *Acupuncture Points Are Holes,* 154, 156, 174; clinic's return on investment, 152; community acupuncture, 144, 145, 147, 148, 151, 155, 174–75; and Liberation Acupuncture, 154, 160–61, 174–75; Monteiro with, 151; perspective on suffering, 174–75, 177; and Phan, 161; POCA Tech, 155; Utah controversy, 158; Working Class Acupuncture, 145–49, 150, 151

Rose City Park United Methodist Church, 158

Rosenberg, Susan, 128, 172

Rosenthal, Mel, 34, 35, 37

Said, Edward, 143, 162

San Francisco Red Guards, 136

scalp acupuncture, 89

Scarlett, Yvonne, 180–81

Schatz, Jean, 116

Scheinberg, Labe, 54

Schmalzer, Sigrid, 28

41–43; methadone maintenance, 59–66; planned shrinkage, 33–39; professionalism, 47–49

Venceremos Brigade, 111
verum acupuncture, 82, 83–84
Vietnam War, 63–64; barefoot medicine practice of, 21; heroin addiction among veterans, 56; veterans, post-traumatic stress disorder in, 59
violence, 129, 154; and conflict, 113; FBI, 131; and healing, 169; nonviolent way, 107, 113, 184; Richard Taft, death, 107; structural, 165

Wallace, Deborah, 35, 38–39, 59
Wallace, Rodrick, 35, 38–39, 59
warming herb, 27
"War on Drugs," 60
WCA (Working Class Acupuncture), 143, 145–49, 150, 151. *See also* POCA
Weatherman, the, 29
Weather Underground Organization, 109, 125
Wen, H. L., 103
Westchester County, 41
Western acupuncture, 81–82, 87, 136, 143, 145
Wexu, Mario, 109, 116–17
Wexu, Oscar, 116–18
Wexus' school, 122, 123
White, Paul Dudley, 19–20
*White Lightning* (newspaper), 95–96
White Lightning, 103–4, 105, 106–7
Williams, Jeral Wayne, 98. *See also* Shakur, Mutulu
Wolpe, Paul Root, 24
World Acupuncture Congress, 119
World Health Organization (WHO), 16–17
Worsley, J. R., 118
Wright, C. R., 63

Young Lords, 15, 50–51, 53, 55, 56, 58, 64–65, 126–127, 154, 168
Yuan-bain, Hong, 136–37

Zeller, Barbara, 59, 109, 110, 113, 117, 118, 124, 125, 131, 134, 189
Zhan, Mei, 8–9, 28–29
Zhiqian, Chen, 145
Zimbabwe African National Union (ZANU), 92, 93